Up
Struggle

Embrace the Struggle

Become Stronger

Live Happier

Tracey Ferrin

WHAT THEY'RE SAYING

"Tracey's message is powerful yet simple. She tells her story with transparency, courage, honesty, and a great sense of humor. Tracey inspires, regardless of race, religion, and gender. We hosted a Women's conference, and Tracey was our keynote, Speaker. She engaged the diverse audience with her testimony." -Alejandro Ezquerra, Author and Pastor

"Tracey Ferrin is a speaker for any occasion in which your group needs inspiration and practical steps for recognizing and conquering "struggles" of any type. Tracey has a personal story that is amazing in its nature; actually, miraculous in her fight and the recovery that she has gone through. All her personal testimony is applied to steps that every audience can see as applicable to their own circumstances. Tracey has a brisk and optimistic way to describe events that should, in every respect, be devastating." -Larry Blair, Vice President, The Rotary Club of the University Area, Houston

"The more I got to know Tracey the more I respected her strength, perseverance, courage, determination, kind heart, and many talents. It's been a delight to see Tracey step into a role as an inspirational leader through public speaking and writing. I believe she was born to shine her light, motivate others, spread positivity, love, and energy." -Ashlie Sustaita, National Fitness Professional & Program Developer

"I am probably the most biased person to write a testimonial, but also by that same standard I am the best since I know her better than anyone else. She is the most authentic, genuine, and inspiring person I know. Her heart is pure, and she passionately motivates and uplifts those around her. Her perspective on life is unlike anyone's I've ever met, she is driven and dedicated to her family, passions, dreams, and her cause. I highly recommend you read her book, connect with her on social media, and be fortunate enough to hear her speak." -Ryan Ferrin, the husband aka: her biggest fan

"Tracey taught me that tough times can help me transform into someone better. She taught me to unapologetically be myself, have fun, and not forget who I am. I love that she does her best to learn from all of the blessings and challenges sent her way. Tracey empowers those around her and loves fiercely." -Krista Grether, friend for over a decade

To the woman who does so much for her family.

Love you, mom!

Contents

I promise, this blank page is here for a reason.

Flip the page to find out why.

Before you continue

I want to share with you how I read my books. When I first started reading, I would only highlight what stood out to me. Then, when I wanted to go back and find that quote I loved, advice I wanted to share, tips to implement into my life, etc. I would find myself spending more time than I wanted trying to find it. "Was it at the beginning? No, it was in the middle next to that one story. No, now I remember, it was definitely at the end. Wait a minute, it wasn't even in this book, it was in the other one!" This is what I'm trying to help you avoid!

Eventually, I got tired of wasting so much time doing this that I came up with a system to help me find the information quicker.

Yes, I still want you to highlight and scribble in this book. But I also want you to use that blank page to write down a few brief words with the page number to the things that stand out to you, so you can easily go back and find it, instead of getting frustrated like I would.

You will also see random blank pages throughout the book. Use them to journal thoughts and impressions.

INTRODUCTION

Ever found yourself in a funk, feeling miserable, suffering, and flat out struggling like I do when I'm trying to take off my sweaty sports bra?

Or maybe you've found yourself saying things like, this sucks! Why me? I don't deserve this. I can't handle this. I've done nothing but make good choices in life. I would give anything to make this go away. I avoid them at all costs. I don't have time for this!

Does any of that sound familiar? I think it's safe to say at some point you have felt this way or said these things about your struggles. Maybe you feel this way right now. Maybe you just said something like this to one of your girlfriends.

I mostly use the word struggle in this book, but what I'm also talking about are things like setbacks, obstacles, trials, challenges, hard times, tribulation, conflict, affliction, adversity, heart ache, pain, or a tough season. All sound like struggles to me.

In this book, you will read about some struggles I have gone through, but also, one very crucial understanding of them.

The understanding? That struggles are for you not against you, if you choose.

Struggles will always be part of the human experience. No one, and I mean no one, is exempt from them.

In fact, at some point in your life (if not already) you will experience a struggle that will down right leave you questioning your faith, your potential, your purpose, and quite frankly, your entire existence.

Along with these struggles I'm going to share with you, I'm also going to share some lessons and tips I've learned from them.

And if some of my words feel like a little kick in the bum, know it's with love.

Some of the struggles I mention in this book will be ones you, a loved one, coworker, or friend have experienced, may be experiencing, or may experience in the future. Others, you may never personally deal with. I have learned that regardless if you experience the exact struggles I have or not, the feelings they can create are very much universal.

Meaning, different struggles can create the same feelings and it's those feelings we can relate to. Different story, same feelings. Why do I think this is important? Because far too often we let the actual struggle itself set us apart from each other. I believe finding common ground with each other is important.

Do you know pain? Great, so do I! We are more alike than you think.

I cannot mention my struggles without mentioning God. One thing I have learned is God often wraps my biggest blessings up and presents them to me as struggles. When I think back on my biggest struggles in life, there too laid my biggest blessings.

In my life, He has been a huge part of helping me get through the hard times. In fact, it's because of Him that I have come to the understanding that struggles are for me. The truth is, it's that understanding that at times is the only thing that has helped me through. Knowing that the struggle is there to help me grow, learn, and give me experience, helps me put one foot in front of the other.

No, you are not the only one who struggles. Although, that is exactly what the adversary would have you believe.

I also look at these struggles as a token of love from God. He knows what I am capable of becoming, but without these struggles, I cannot become that person.

Growth wasn't designed to take place in comfort. We must allow ourselves to get uncomfortable in life. Getting uncomfortable takes place on so many levels, but we don't have to be in constant pain to grow. We just need some resistance. And when you find it, don't rush it, stay in it and allow change to take place.

Now, if you're thinking you are going to read about how graceful I was during my struggles, how I never doubted my faith, or that I didn't stumble, fall, and even play in the mud before getting back up, that couldn't be further from the truth.

Because the truth is, most often than not, I struggled big, fell hard, and sometimes I rolled around in the mud so long before getting back up that it started to stain my skin. Can mud even stain your skin? I don't know, but if it can, it certainly did mine.

Just because I am writing this book doesn't mean I am perfect at any of what you are fixing to read about or that I don't still struggle at times to use my own advice, because sometimes I totally do. Yes, I am teaching you what I have learned, but I am first and foremost a student of these teachings.

Writing this book does mean that I am willing to get over myself enough to share some hard things I've gone through with you. Plus, what I have discovered along the way and what has helped me.

I look at each struggle I learn from like adding a tool to my toolbox.

Who wants a toolbox with just a screwdriver? Not me! Try fixing everything in life with that. Each tool I earn (because they are definitely earned) helps me grow as a person. The more tools I have, the better equipped I am to handle the next struggle that comes my way.

You see, I believe we all have superpowers. One of mine? Using my struggles as growth opportunities. This too can become one of your superpowers!

I never imagined I would be able to write a book. Nothing in my past says I would be an author or a motivational speaker. Nothing! Yet here I am.

This book wasn't written overnight. It took me 18 years to write this book. Without my cancer, the people who had a hand in saving my life, all my struggles along the way, and the lessons I've learned, this book would not be possible.

Having had cancer was the worst thing I have ever experienced. To date, it was the hardest struggle I have ever been through. But if I could go back and change it, I wouldn't. I took way too much from that experience. It added value beyond measure to my life.

My belief system about struggles didn't come overnight. It started off as a small flame and with each struggle, I was able to fuel that flame to the size of a bonfire! I'm talking TEXAS size! #gobigorgohome

I don't have these beliefs about struggles just because they make me feel better. Although they do. I have these beliefs because I have personally experienced what I'm sharing in this book for myself. And I know if these things help me the way they do, they too can help you. This isn't something that only works for a select few, either. This works for anyone willing to put it to work.

Although I still have struggles in my life, I am far better able to get through them and put them to work for me. It really is about the beliefs and mindset we have going into a struggle that makes all the difference.

I've learned that struggles are universal experiences, but what's not universal is what people *choose* to believe about them and what they *choose* to do with them.

I'm just a Texas girl, who realized she could let her struggles take from her, or she could take from them.

My wish for you, sweet friend, is that you will learn to take from your struggles instead of allowing them to take from you. That you will search, seek, hunt, and yes, sometimes even have to dig for the lesson. But I promise, if you do, you will find it. In this book, I will teach you how.

Navigating through a struggle will take work. Sister, I'm here for you, but I can't do the work for you. That part is on you.

So, lean in, open your heart and mind, be intentional in your reading, commit to flipping each page, highlight what stands out to you, scribble impressions, doggie ear pages, ponder, and become a believer with me, that the struggle is for you not against you, if you choose.

Xo, Tracey

Hang on sister, this struggle is going to take you on a ride of a lifetime.

#upstruggle

Chapter 1
Biggest struggle of my life

When I was 18, I was diagnosed with Osteosarcoma. Also known as bone cancer, a rare cancer, targets the young cancer, and totally sucks cancer. I mean, let's be real, I guess any kind of cancer sucks, right?

Did you know that roughly 16,000 cases of childhood cancer are diagnosed each year, and that's just in the United States? And out of 16,000 cases, approximately 450 will be childhood osteosarcoma. Crazy, right?

Oh, I forgot to mention that when I was diagnosed with this cancer, I was also 6 months pregnant, married, and had a 10-month-old daughter. Go ahead, pick your jaw up from the ground. I know, it sounds like a lot to deal with, and it most certainly was.

Having had this cancer already put me in rare category. Throwing pregnancy on top of it made it an even more difficult case to treat.

My Oncologist advised me to terminate my pregnancy. He said they didn't have any research showing a healthy baby being born to a mother who underwent chemo in her 1st or 2nd trimester.

I told my doctor that termination wasn't an option and that chemo would have to wait until after she was born. He told me waiting wasn't an option. By then it could be too late.

You see, I had high-grade osteosarcoma, meaning it grows and spreads quickly if left untreated. The problem with this is depending on if and where it spread, it could make treating me harder and lower my 5-year survival rate from 60-80 % to as low as 15-30%.

No matter how young a mother is, her instinct to protect her child is fierce.

All I could think about was saving my unborn child's life. All my doctor was thinking about was saving mine.

Now, my doctor meant well. He is a sweet old man that holds a special place in my heart. He was only advising what he thought was best for me as his patient. I understood where he was coming from but also knew I was the one who had to live with the decision.

What I heard him say through the fog of it all was I had to choose between my daughter who was already born and the one living and growing inside me.

Because choosing Elly meant losing my unborn child and choosing my unborn child meant losing my life and neither of my girls having a mother to raise them.

It was up to me to make an impossible decision. How was I ever going to choose? How could any mother be expected to make that kind of decision? Especially a mother as young as I was. The decision rested solely on my shoulders.

It's not that the decision to keep my unborn child was hard. That was actually very easy. Because one thing I knew was that little girl inside of me would live no matter the cost. The hard part? Making sure there were 3 lives at the end of it all. How was I going to make sure those two little girls got to keep their mom?

Thankfully, I'm stubborn and a fighter. Or, as my dad would call me, hardheaded. Either way, it played in my favor.

Tell me no, tell me I can't, tell me it's impossible, try and place your limitations on me, and I will prove you wrong every time. Yes, it's a twisted need of mine. But it actually fuels me and drives me to accomplish the things I set out to do, especially when others tell me I can't.

With me not budging on termination, it forced my doctor to come up with another plan. He told me that if I waited until my third trimester to start chemo, my daughter would have a good shot at survival but that he couldn't give me any guarantees as to what chemo might do to her.

After talking this through with my mother, I agreed to the new treatment plan. Thankfully, I was only 3 weeks away from my third trimester. Although he wanted to start chemo right away, waiting 3 weeks seemed far better than 3 months.

It seemed like the only logical way to give all 3 of us a fighting chance to be standing together at the end of everything we were fixing to endure. This meant I was taking some risk, but so was my unborn child. Was it ideal? No. But it seemed like the only way.

This meant Elly had her mother, my unborn child would live, and I was going to be able to raise my girls. In my heart, I knew my baby would be ok! That knowledge is what allowed me to move forward with this new plan of action.

After the 3-week waiting period, I was scheduled to be admitted to MD Anderson Cancer Center (MDACC) on 9/11/2001. Yes, that was the day that our country stood still. The day that our country and so many lives changed forever. The day we were under attack. And the day we will never forget.

Due to those horrific events, my chemo was delayed to the next day. While the world was glued to their TV screens and our country was preparing to go to war, I too was under attack, preparing for the biggest battle of my life.

I brought in my first round of chemo like a champ. I even shaved my head. I was told I would lose my hair due to the chemo, so I figured instead of waiting around for it to fall out and feeling like it was taken from me, I would do it myself.

My first round of chemo seemed to go pretty well. I even remember thinking, "Why is everyone taking this cancer thing so seriously? It's not even that big of a deal, I feel great. If this is what chemo is like, bring on the chemo! I got this!"

Oh, little did I know. Little did I know that with each round of chemo, my body would get weaker. Little did I know what was waiting right around the corner.

After that first round of chemo was complete, my husband left me. When we informed the staff at MDACC, they said that was actually quite normal and that more men leave their wives when they get sick than women leave their husbands.

I hold no ill feelings towards him. Although at the time, I was extremely heartbroken. His family told me he couldn't stand by and watch the girl he loved die.

Even though I kind of grasped that, it didn't make me feel any better. He was also young, and I know expecting him to care for me was asking a lot of him. He did the best he could under a horrible circumstance. I filed for a divorce.

I was already living with my parents. It was agreed that my husband would care for me and our daughter and my parents would work. Now what was I supposed to do?

My sister Porscha ended up coming home to take care of my daughter. My mom ended up getting fired because she missed so much work taking care of me and getting me to and from the hospital. And my dad continued to work. Saying this situation was far from ideal and put a strain on everyone, is an understatement. But it became our new normal. My family was determined to help me fight this disease, no matter the cost. I am forever grateful to them for all they did for me and my girls.

After doing 2 more rounds of chemo with my daughter, she was born 6 weeks early. My Doctor wanted to take her as early as possible without having any major complications from being a preemie.

I knew I was in good hands; my High Risk OBGYN was an amazing doctor, and I fully trusted him with the life of my unborn child. (He's also the doctor who delivered the sextuplets back in April 2015 from the TV show, Out Daughtered.)

There I was, as bald as Mr. Clean, giving birth to a 3 lbs. 10 oz. screaming baby girl with a head full of dark brown hair! The doctors, my family, and I all took this as a good sign. We knew this meant she was a fighter and was going to be ok. I named her Fayth Marie.

While Fayth stayed in the NICU for a few weeks, putting some meat on her bones, I headed back to the purple floors of MDACC to finish one more round of chemo before having to endure the 13-hour limb salvage surgery. Yes, just how it sounds. A surgery to save my leg.

Christmas was fast approaching, and I was still in the hospital recovering from this surgery. The doctors didn't think I would make it home for Christmas, but I assured them I would. They thought I didn't understand what they were telling me. I understood them clearly. They didn't understand me. I told them, "With or without your permission, I am leaving this hospital so I can spend Christmas at home with my two girls." Yes, I was "that" kind of patient. It was going to be Fayth's first Christmas, and I was not going to miss it.

5

Reluctantly, I was released Christmas morning!

We brought in the new year with more chemo and all the side effects imaginable. 2002 was where things started getting tricky. It was hands down one of the hardest years of my life.

Each chemo presented its own set of side effects. I dealt with kidney failure and mouth sores so painful I could barely eat or drink, which led to extreme weight loss and dehydration, which landed me back at MDACC emergency room.

But when I did feel up to eating or drinking, Taco Bell and red fruit punch was my go-to. I would not recommend that diet to anyone, under any circumstance, especially someone who is as sick as I was. Many years later, my mom and I had a pretty good laugh about the fact that she didn't appreciate all the red stains on the carpet from all the times I couldn't make it to a toilet or bowl to throw up.

I dealt with low blood counts, which led to receiving multiple blood transfusions that made me feel like a new woman! Secretly hoping that every time they ran my blood work, they would say I needed a blood transfusion, that's how good they made me feel. I was like, bring on the blood!

I was overdosed on a chemo called Methotrexate which led to waking up one day without the use of my motor skills. Talk about scary! I didn't know if this was going to be the new me. There I was, once again at MDACC emergency room.

They brought in a neurologist to try and figure out what was wrong with me. You know those cards you show your toddler when you are trying to teach them something new? The ones with shapes, colors, and objects. Those were the cards he was showing me. He asked me if I knew what they were.

I knew that I knew what he was showing me, but I wasn't able to communicate it to him because I couldn't speak. So, he then had to find another approach in trying to figure out if I knew what he was showing me. I ended up nodding yes if what he said was correct and no if what he told me was incorrect. In the end, all they had to do was double me up on some meds that helped my body clear the chemo quicker.

I couldn't walk by myself due to the surgery. Crutches it was, independence gone, frustration started to build. I even remember this one time I was using 1 crutch to hobble around. All I wanted to do was get my own glass of water. I mean, I just wanted some sense of independence.

I realized that using 1 crutch would give me that independence I needed. I ended up falling and crying so hard that I couldn't catch my breath. My mom rushed over to me to see if I was ok and if I had hurt or damaged my leg. Thankfully, my leg was fine. I had no physical pain from the fall. It was emotional pain being released. It was the straw that broke the camel's back, and I completely lost it.

From the isolation of being in the hospital and the toll all of this was taking on me, I slipped into a depression, and, at that time in my life, the only way I knew how to deal with it was to use my pain meds I was prescribed from my leg surgery. And let me tell you, my doctor was liberal in giving me pain meds. 100 pill bottles with my name all over them, and I wasn't complaining. If I wasn't in physical pain, I was in mental and emotional pain. Taking those pills transported me to a place of feeling carefree and not having to face my reality.

Towards the end of treatment, I eventually got to the point that I felt like death would be better than what I was going through. It wasn't that I truly wanted to die, but it seemed like a better alternative than my current situation. I was tired of being tired, I was tired of being in pain, and I was tired of suffering. There were definitely moments that if death was a painless option, I might have taken it.

I remember this one day my mom came into my room to give me my pills and I told her no. I told her to just let me die because I couldn't take it any longer. There I was, a mother of two little girls, in the ring with cancer, taking hit after hit and trying my very best to not lose the fight, for them.

What I failed to see was I too was someone's daughter, and she was going to fight to make sure I was around to not just be her daughter but the mother of those two little girls. The look in her eyes that day when I told her no and to just let me die said, "With or without your permission, you will take these pills."

I knew she meant business. My mom is a strong woman, and I knew that if I could no longer fight for myself, she would fight for me. And that is exactly what she did. I wasn't alone in that ring, even though often times I felt like I was. She was there the whole time taking the hits with me. She held me up when I could no longer stand by myself. She helped me win that fight.

My body was shutting down, and I knew if I completed those few last rounds of chemo my doctor had scheduled, I would die. The cancer wasn't killing me. The chemo slowly was! I knew it. My spirit knew it. I could feel it in my bones.

I was again faced with another difficult decision. Either end chemo and take the risk of my cancer not being completely gone or continue on with the treatment plan and surely die. While thinking about what to do, I thought about my uncle who had leukemia and passed away about 10 years earlier.

And I knew if I finished those last few rounds of chemo, my outcome would be the same as my Uncle's. Roughly 14 months after being told I had cancer; I decided no more!!

Use what you went
through to help
someone get through.

#upstruggle

Chapter 2
Not for nothing

You could say going to war with cancer beat me up pretty good, that's a fair statement. But I am here writing this book today because I won that battle, and I even have the scars to prove it! Oh, do I have the scars.

You know, I truly thought my life would go back to normal. Well, at least that's what I was hoping for. Something I didn't understand, and I think a lot of people don't understand, is just because treatments are done or you are cancer free, means life goes back to the way it was before, or that it should.

My experience with cancer was very traumatic and life altering. I needed to allow my body that I had just poisoned for over a year time to heal along with my heart and mind.

I had to relearn how to walk, which was a long and painful process. I'm happy to announce, I no longer walk with a limp! Well, some days I do, days when my leg hurts. Which isn't often.

I had to step back into a world that I was no longer familiar with because when I was sick, I couldn't be in public or around anyone with the slightest sniffle. My life consisted of my bed and MD Anderson.

I couldn't speak about what I had just gone through, to the point that I would get upset if anyone I knew talked about it in front of me or asked me questions. I so badly wanted to brush it under a rug, act like it never happened, and move on with my life.

Out of sight out of mind, right?

But here's what I've learned about brushing things under the rug: They may be out of sight, but until properly dealt with, will also be that ugly lump under the rug that you constantly trip over.

11

My mom kept telling me that I needed to talk about what I had been through. I believe the words that came out of her mouth were something like this, "Tracey, the more you talk about your experience, the better you will feel." And I believe my dad's words were something like this, "Your experience can help so many people, you need to share it."

Does anyone else know more than their parents in their early 20s or was that just me? Insert sarcasm.

I was like, "First of all, woman, you just need to be quiet." Not that I actually said that to her because if you know my mom, you know that wouldn't fly. But I was thinking it! I was also thinking, "Well, it's my story, and it's easy to say I should share it when it's not your story." Although, it is very much my parents' story too.

But really, I just nodded while my parents would say this, while thinking those things in my head and silently rolling my eyes.

I could never quite shake their advice, though. With time, I started sharing bits and pieces of my story with others. I'm talking small bits and pieces. As I would do this, I realized that pile under the rug got smaller. I felt better, and I felt like I was on the road to proper recovery. Until I was able to embrace my own story, I wasn't able to share it. It really is true, the more you talk about the hard things, the less power they have over you and the better you feel. And in the process of healing, you get to help others as well.

So, I guess my parents were on to something! I mean, you don't actually think I'm going to say they were right, do you? Let's just keep that little secret between you and me for now....wink wink.

I was never that person who said, "Why me?"

My focus was to simply endure my struggle, so when it ended, I could move on. At least the person asking, "Why me?" is truly seeking some kind of understanding. I didn't care to understand. I just wanted to get out of the discomfort as quickly as possible.

I always heard there is light at the end of the tunnel, so I knew if I held on long enough, it would eventually show itself. The part I failed to recognize was I only see that light if I actually move towards it. Moving towards it takes work. If the work isn't done, you move from one dark tunnel to the next.

The Up Struggle Formula

I've been through a lot. Cancer was just my ultimate struggle. After everything I had been through, I wanted to believe it wasn't for nothing and that good really could come from it.

One day, I decided it was time to really dive into understanding struggles. The way I did this was through reflection of my own struggles and the good ole Google search bar.

The idea that struggles could be for me instead of against me was born. This idea led to my perception of struggles. My perception led to my belief. And my belief has led to how I deal with them.

Through it all, I came to an understanding that struggles really weren't the enemy. Struggles were growth opportunities in disguise. No matter how big or small the struggle is, each one has value to offer, but I knew it was up to me to find the value and then apply it to my life.

Through all the reflection and use of that Google search bar, I discovered there were 3 types of universal struggles. Now, when I say universal, I mean it doesn't matter the make and model of the car you drive, how big your home is, what your bank statement says, what titles you hold, or what family you were born into. Everyone will experience struggles from these 3 categories.

The first one I call SELF, meaning: self-inflicted pain by one's own actions. Ouch, right! Who wants to hear that?

Some struggles are so painful that we never repeat them, but what about the ones that repeat over and over? Repeated struggles fall under self. A repeated struggle is what I like to call feedback. Feedback that in order to stop repeating it, you must change your actions. Because it's your actions that keep it on repeat mode in the first place. So, it's your actions that will get you off it. This can only take place if you are willing to accept responsibility for your choices.

Remember how in the intro to this book, I told you some of my words may feel like a little kick in the bum? Well, if it felt that way, that is what I like to call feedback too, and I would listen to it.

Chin up, sister, the good news is, now that you know this, you can work on it. Whereas before, you couldn't because you simply weren't aware of it. And if you were, this is just a friendly reminder to keep working on this. Trust me, I was this girl for so many years, and if I can work on it, so can you.

The second one I call OTHERS, meaning: pain inflicted on you due to the actions of others. Now, this is usually where we want to place most our struggles, but let's be real, most of them don't belong here, and if you think they do, the question now becomes, why are you surrounding yourself with people who don't value you and only cause you pain?

If you feel like most of your struggles fall into this category, then really, they actually fall under SELF.

Because you are allowing this to happen. Again, ouch! But friend, sometimes the truth hurts and doesn't feel good. Doesn't make it any less true. But because I care, I am willing to tell you some hard things.

The third one I call LIFE, meaning: pain inflicted on you at no one's fault. Like my cancer and hurricane Harvey.

These struggles, well, you just have to roll with the punches. I call this category "life" for a reason. Because neither you nor someone else has control over having these struggles.

Here are some questions I ask myself to help me figure out which category my struggle falls under.

1. Did I bring this upon myself? If so, what can I do differently to avoid it in the future? A little taste of humble pie and a willingness to take accountability is needed to ask this one. (Definitely ask this when a struggle is on repeat.)

   I'm not talking about a cheating husband. There is never an excuse for that. I'm not talking about an abusive family member. Don't you let them tell you it was your fault because you didn't force them to do it. So, don't you dare let other people put that on you. And don't you dare put that on yourself. You don't get to take responsibility for that one. You do get to take responsibility for what you choose to do moving forward, though. What you choose to do moving forward can be empowering!

   What I'm talking about here is more along the lines of a falling out with a friend, miscommunication, getting fired, hurt feelings, etc.

2. Did someone else bring this upon me? If so, what actions are needed?

   I have found that often times 3 actions are needed for this one:

   • I need to put a little distance between myself and the other person.

   • I need to have a conversation with them about what is and isn't acceptable in my life.

   • I need to set clearer boundaries.

Because this I know, I can't get mad at someone who has crossed one of my boundaries if I never made that boundary clear to begin with. I mean, I guess I could get mad, but what good is that going to do for the situation?

3. If I answer no to questions 1 and 2, then it falls into the Life category.

You may not always have control over having struggles in your life, but you can certainly choose to focus on the controllables. Is controllables even a word? Because word doc isn't recognizing it as one. Squirrel!

Meaning, what you do have control over, put your focus and energy on those things. And those things would be how you choose to respond to your struggles and what you choose to believe about them.

Hey, I get it! Not always easy. This takes some practice for sure. It's like any other habit, it takes time to develop. Be patient with yourself and know this will become a part of who you are the more you do it. It's ok if it feels weird at first, that too will go away with time and practice.

I have also come up with some reminders that help me when I'm struggling.

1. You are not meant to go through this alone. Who are you leaning on that is helping you get through this?

I want you to take a minute to think about a person or persons that you turn to when you are struggling. If you can't come up with anyone, this is a problem. Often times, we want to isolate ourselves when things get hard. But that is absolutely the last thing you want to do. That only makes things worse.

Why do we wait till things are really hard and we are suffocating before leaning on others? Why do we wait till the divorce papers have been filed to tell others about the divorce? By the time the papers are filed, extreme pain has been endured. I believe we do this because we don't want to be a burden to others, we think that what we are going through is nothing compared to our other friend, or we feel shame.

I have learned that people want to help, and they love being asked. It shows you trust them enough to confide in them. I mean, just think back to a time someone came to you with something personal. Didn't it make you feel really good that someone would seek you out or think highly enough of you that they would talk to you about some hard things?

It doesn't matter what your other friend is going through. Just because her struggle seems harder than yours doesn't mean you aren't allowed to struggle with the thing you are dealing with. Now hear me loud and clear, no one gets to tell you if your struggle is hard or easy. Your easy could be my hard. My easy could be your hard. It's all relative to the individual and their own experience, knowledge, environment, and support system. You and I could have the same struggle and experience it differently. That's ok!

And as far as shame, you are not your struggle. It is merely an experience you are having. You can't be divorce. You can't be abuse. You can't be cancer. You can't be bankruptcy. You can be human, though; I mean, you are that.

Here are a few examples of who you can lean on: your partner, God, friends, family, church leader. Anyone you trust falls into this category.

2.   Do things you know that will lift your spirit.

When I was giving a speech and I asked that as a question, a man shouted out, "costumes!"

You see, this man's wife was undergoing chemotherapy at MDACC. And every time she did chemo, she would dress up as a superhero. After my speech, he showed me a few pictures of his wife dressed up in her costumes.

I thought that was a neat idea! For his wife, it made her feel better. Keep in mind, what makes one person feel better may not work for another person, and that's ok.

I want to share with you some things I do that might help you come up with some of your own ideas, if you are feeling a bit lost with this one.

I personally enjoy moving my body! AKA: exercise. Moving my body always helps me feel better. Now, moving my body and moving your body can look totally different. But moving the body is for everyone. It's like not even an opinion, it's a fact. Google it, because we know that if Google says so, it's true.

Maybe you like to go on long runs. Me – no thank you! I'm that friend who will hop on her bike if you insist that I go on a run with you. Because this girl has never been a fan of running, like ever. But this doesn't mean it's not good for you or that it won't make you feel better. It just means it doesn't make me feel better, actually quite the opposite.

Maybe you like taking a spin class? Maybe you like to shake what your mama gave you with Zumba? Maybe you're like Gumby (if you don't know who Gumby is, you are way too young to be reading this book) and enjoy Yoga? If you don't like to move your body, it's only because you haven't found what kind of movement you like. So sister, try them all! Try as many styles you can get your hands on or until you find something that sticks. Something that gets you out of bed. Something that you are excited to do. Just move your body. Preferably 3-5 times a week. Daily if you can!

I also like to read books! You know what's crazy? Just a few short years ago, I was a girl who hated reading.

Now, I'm not someone who uses the word hate lightly. Like I don't even say that in reference to people. Because I believe hating someone is wrong on so many levels. No, that was not me waving my Christian girl flag. That was me waving my Personal Development flag.

I mean, I thought people who read books were just wasting their time. I'm so dead serious. Yet, here I am writing a book just 4 short years after I started reading them. Oh, how things can take a complete 180.

I also love podcasts! My favorite one right now is the Empower HER podcast hosted by Kacia Fitzgerald. Now, she is a woman who gets life and tells it in real time! Her superpower is having the ability to see the silver lining in everything.

She is all about taking purpose driven action toward building the life she really freaking loves. In her podcast, she shares stories, tips, and tricks to help you get out of your own way and unapologetically make some moves. You should go check her out on the podcast app. No doubt you will love her as much as I do. And if you slide into her DM's, tell her I sent you.

How about 89.3 KSBJ? KSBJ is a radio station that plays upbeat modern Christian music to Houston and beyond. I just love that they are a clean radio station that's all about serving people. Be it with uplifting music that will get to your feels and maybe even make you shed a tear or two or running a fundraiser to help give back to the community.

Ok, will most definitely make you shed a tear or two to the point that if you're wearing makeup, just forget about it not getting ruined. Because it will. There is no pretty crying when it comes to KSBJ. And

I don't mean crying in a bad way but more like in a therapeutic way. A way that is cleansing for the soul. Not that I know from experience or anything...

These are a few things that lift my spirit when I'm feeling down or struggling. Oh, I've got a few more really quick. Food, a shower, and a clean home, all help me feel better! Just had to throw those in there because they really do help. My husband knows when I'm struggling to make sure my belly is fed, my house is clean, and I've showered for the day. Because who wants to be around a stinky struggling hungry mama – no one!

Maybe these things will help you too. But if not, that's ok.

Maybe for you it's hanging out with friends, watching a movie, doing cartwheels, snuggling your cat or dog, drinking a nice warm cup of honey lemon water, but whatever it is, as long as it's adding value to your life and making you feel better, do more of it. Especially when you are struggling.

If you drink alcohol, definitely do not do more of that. Struggles and alcohol are not a good mix, and I can hear you now, "But Tracey, you said do more of the thing that makes me feel better." Yes, but not that. That will only mask your issue when you should be facing it. That is not adding value to your life. That is only temporarily making you feel better about a situation that alcohol cannot make go away.

Again, think back to the last few times you were struggling. What did you do that made you feel better?

Write them down below.

1.

2.

3.

4.

5.

6.

7.

8.

9.

10.

And if you're not sure what makes you feel better, keep searching and trying new things. You could always ask some friends what they do and try those things too. Or ask them what they have seen you do that makes you happy.

3. This is for you not against you, if you choose. So, lean in and search for the lesson it has to offer. I believe deep down we all know the lessons we need to learn, and if we are going to learn them, we need to be primed for them. What this means is pride and ego have to be placed aside

Leading with those things will only prevent you from learning the things you need to learn. It's imperative that you are primed for learning.

Glass of humble juice anyone? Being humble does not mean beating yourself up or belittling yourself either, so don't head down that rabbit hole. Being humble means, you are willing to look in the mirror and accept the truth that you do have a hand in some of your struggles.

4. This will make you stronger! I mean, put that on repeat like you do a Kane Brown song. Play it like a broken record. Over and over and over until you truly believe it. Sometimes when I'm having a hard time, this and #7 are the only things that help me. Struggles

are meant to change you but how will always be up to you. You can let it make you bitter or make you better. Whichever one you choose is a choice.

5. Remember that one time you got through that really difficult trial in your life, when you wanted to give up but didn't? You got this, girl! A little pep talk can go a long way. I don't need to know you personally to know that if you are reading this book, you have been through some stuff. Yet here you are! How could I possibly know this? Because you are human, and remember, no one is exempt from struggles. No one.

For me, being able to identify my hardest struggle has been a blessing. I use it as a reference point for all the other challenging times in my life.

It reminds me that if I could get through cancer, then I can get through anything. Yes, it's true, one day I may find myself in a struggle that is harder than cancer. But even then, I know I will get through it one way or another because I know I can do hard things. Having cancer showed me that. Take a moment to identify your "cancer." Maybe you too can use it as a reminder of just how strong you really are.

List your "cancer" below.

_____

6. Focus on the solution to the struggle. What you focus on, you will always get more of. I want you to stare at one thing that is in the room with you. Like hard core focus on it. Notice anything? Everything else around what you are focusing on becomes blurry. When literally right next to your struggle could be the solution to it, but because you are so focused on the struggle instead of the solution, you get more struggle.

7. Use what you went through to help someone get through. I think that one is pretty straight forward. I mean, what's even the point of learning something if we aren't going to share it with others?

I believe that learning things and then keeping it all to myself is quite selfish. If I can shorten someone's learning curve or someone can learn from my struggles, I'm all in.

I've noticed something about sharing lessons I've learned from struggles. When I teach what I know, I know what I teach. It becomes more ingrained into my beliefs and flows out of me easier. So really, by helping others, I am also solidifying my own beliefs.

All the reminders I have shared, you may not use all at once. Some you may find more helpful than others in certain struggles. I didn't share them with an expectation that you would use all of them every time you struggle. I shared them because I wanted to provide you with enough tools to choose from. Choose away!

I learned that when life felt hard, I needed to recognize it as a struggle so that I could apply my knowledge to them. We can't work on what we don't acknowledge. We also can't work on what we don't embrace. Embracing a struggle does not mean we have to be happy about it, but it does mean we accept it. Can I get an AMEN up in here!

So, once you recognize and embrace it as a struggle, you can now move into reflection. Here, you can identify which universal struggle it is you're dealing with by asking those questions I shared with you earlier in this chapter. In case you already forgot, here they are again. 1. Did I bring this upon myself? 2. Did someone else bring this upon me? 3. Answering no to both those questions means it falls under Life.

Whether we reflect in the struggle or out of it, what matters most is that at some point, we reflect.

The smaller struggles are easier to reflect in, and the harder ones are easier to reflect out of or at least once the fog starts to lift. As long as you reflect, the struggle doesn't go to waste. The struggle isn't using you, but you are now using it.

Through all this reflection and being primed to learn, a lesson or two or more are born. Then we move into applying the lesson to our lives. This is where the magic really takes place. Because without this, we can't move forward.

When we apply the lessons to our lives, it simply means we are growing as human beings. And isn't that what life is all about, or at least a huge part of it? Progressing on our journey. Knowing better so we can do better so we can become better.

Growth equals progress. And for me and everyone I know, progress equals happiness. Is your mind blown like mine was when I stumbled across this revelation?! Sister, happiness is the end result when this formula is worked. Broken down it looks like this.

Struggle + Reflection = Lesson

Applied Lesson = Growth

Growth = Progress

Progress = Happiness

Simply put...

Struggle

=

Happiness

I know what you're thinking. "She's crazy, run!" You aren't the only one.

You know, chemo did give me 1 very cool superpower. That superpower? Reading minds. And what I hear when I explain this to people is 2 things:

1. Get the pitchforks, she has done lost her mind! Who brought her here to speak to us?

2. Huh? Now that's a belief I can stand behind.

We like number two.

Psychology 101

Have you ever heard of confirmation bias? Confirmation bias just means that you look for evidence to confirm your beliefs. As humans, we do this with everything.

If we are going to look for evidence to confirm our beliefs, why not make sure our beliefs are empowering us, serving us, and beneficial? The beliefs you and I have are a choice. Knowing this, it's time to let go of some old beliefs that do not serve you and create new ones that do.

Take a minute to think about 3 limiting beliefs. A limiting belief is a belief that is not serving you. AKA: unkind thoughts that hold you back in life. List them below.

Example: ***Old belief:* I'm not a good mom.**

1.

2.

3.

Now I want you to create 3 new beliefs that you are going to replace those old beliefs with, that you know will serve you. List them below.

Example: *New belief:* **I'm a great mom.**

1.

2.

3.

Now think of any supporting evidence you can use to support your new beliefs. If you can't think of something, go to a trusted source and ask them to help you. Your supporting evidence is tailored and personal to you.

Supporting Evidence: I love my kids. I serve them. I spend time with them. I set boundaries. I tell them no. I encourage them. I let them do hard things. We laugh together. I would die for them. Etc.

1.

2.

3.

Examples of different kinds of supporting evidence

Old belief: Why bother working out, I never stick with it anyway.

Negative Supporting Evidence to the old belief may sound like this in your head, "You can't do it, remember that one time you signed up for a gym membership and then never used it? Or that one time you started your own health and fitness business and it didn't work out? Yeah, don't even try. You're such a failure."

New belief: I want to start working out so I can feel better about myself.

Positive Supporting Evidence to a new belief may sound like this in your head, "You can do it, remember that one time you trained for a half marathon and then totally owned it? Or that one year you woke up at 4:30 am for an entire year just so you could get your run in before you left for work. What about that season you coached soccer and did all the workouts with the girls? Oh girl, you got this! Doesn't mean it will be easy, but you can do hard things."

Give yourself some grace if you don't get it right the first several times. Heck, if you're anything like me, maybe the first 1,000 times you try this you will suck at it, but if you don't give up, it will become a new way of life for you. It will take being intentional with your thoughts. You will start to notice that finding positive supporting evidence to new beliefs that serve you will start to make you feel better about yourself.

Keep in mind, the work is the same no matter which belief (limiting or serving) you have or supporting evidence (negative or positive) you look for. The kind that builds you up or the kind that knocks you down. The kind that will give you confidence to do the things or the kind that will zap it. The kind that adds to your trust bucket or the kind that takes away. So, why not choose the supporting evidence that makes you feel better?

Let your struggle launch you into something better.

#upstruggle

Chapter 3
Hope Floats

After my divorce was final, I knew I wanted to step back into the dating scene. Being divorced meant I had the freedom to mingle with the young single adults in my church and open myself up to the possibility of love. Off I went to my first activity. It was 2003 and around Halloween. I remember because I went to an activity where we were decorating pumpkins and the weather was cooler.

This man that I had briefly been introduced to a week or so before, came up to me and asked me what my name was, again. I said, "My name is Tracey. And I remember your name, Ryan." I then walked off.

I knew that was him trying to play it cool or act like I didn't leave some kind of impression on him the first time we met. I, for one, wasn't into playing games. Off I went to enjoy time with my friends for the remainder of the evening.

A few days later, I was with a group of church friends at a Denny's restaurant, and as we were leaving to go home, that guy Ryan showed up and said, "If anyone needs a ride home, I can take you." I looked at him and said, "If you want to take me home, just ask."

So, he did, and I let him take me home. I didn't find out until later that sealed the deal for him. A woman who was direct was just what he liked.

I was invited to attend a young single adult dance. As I sat on one of those cold metal chairs, some random guy sat by me and was trying to pick me up. I didn't care too much for his company, and I knew with every fiber in my being that him and I were not going to be a thing. I guess you could say that it was probably written all over my face that I wasn't feeling it with him.

Next thing I know, that guy Ryan, who asked me what my name was again and took me home from Denny's, sat down next to me and put his arm around me. Not only was I slightly relieved, I thought to myself, "This guy has got some balls!" I was intrigued.

The other man then got up and left. Ryan asked me to dance, and I said yes because I wanted to get to know this man who just got me out from an uncomfortable situation, but who also exhibited a level of confidence I didn't often see. Confidence that I found attractive.

As we were dancing, one of the very first things I told him was that I was recently divorced with two little girls. I wasn't into playing games nor was I going to hide that part of my life. And if I'm being totally honest, after what he had just done, I wanted to see how he would respond to that kind of information. He didn't skip a beat. We danced and talked till the song was over.

Later that evening, he offered to take me (Did I forget to mention he brought one girl to the dance but left with another?) home, and on the way home, he got us lost. Well, that's what he claimed anyway. I believed he just wanted to spend more time with me, and he thought getting us lost would accomplish that. And it did! We talked the entire time and got to know each other a bit better.

When he dropped me off, we exchanged phones numbers and he asked me out on an official date. He said the single adults were going to Galveston for a bonfire and he wanted me to go with him. I was excited!

At the bonfire, there was music, so naturally, he asked me to dance. I mean, what girl doesn't want to dance on the beach with a hot guy? It was straight out of a movie scene, sister!

I couldn't believe what my heart and hands were feeling. My heart felt connected to his. My hands felt all the muscle under his clothes that he was not showing off! I was in complete shock that under his long sleeve shirt were rock solid arms. Like why isn't this guy flaunting his body!?

Then it happened – he asked me if he could kiss me. I was thinking, "Dude, you just ruined the moment and made it awkward." But of course, I still said yes. I will never forget this moment, I literally had to interrupt our kissing sesh and take control of it. All I can say is juicy peach. That's what it was like kissing that man for the very first time. I guess that perfect movie scene had to stop at some point, right?

I came to realize that as confident as he was, it wasn't the "look at me confidence," it was more along the lines of a silent humble confidence. Which is why he didn't flaunty his body, although he had every right to, and I most certainly would have appreciated it. I also realized that him asking if he could kiss me was his way of showing me respect.

That night, after he dropped me off at home, I told my mom I was going to marry him! I just knew it, and I was claiming it. After that night, we were inseparable. If we weren't hanging out, we were on the phone together. Then he met my girls, it was such a natural relationship for my girls and him. Nothing ever felt forced and nothing ever was.

Four weeks after meeting, Ryan asked me to marry him! I said yes. Then, I actually tried to break it off with him. I started to let fear creep into my mind and heart. I started to focus on the two totally different worlds we came from.

Ryan was in school, had ambition, had goals, was an Eagle Scout, never once touched drugs or alcohol, saved himself for his future wife (aka virgin), seemed to make all the right choices, came from a home where his parents were still married, church goer his whole life, served a two year mission for our church, and just seemed to have everything going for him.

Here I was, broken, trying to get my life back on track, just finished fighting cancer a year before, recently divorced, teen mom, made so many mistakes, and thought a girl like me didn't deserve a guy like him.

I was also scared of getting my heart broken again. He seemed too good to be true that I thought surely this would all end once we got married and he let his true colors shine through. And then, I would feel stuck in a marriage that I wasn't happy in. Or somehow, I would screw it up. I mean, who gets engaged after only 4 weeks of knowing each other?! And what's the probability of it even working out?!

I'll tell you who – his parents. His father proposed to his mother after 3 weeks of dating and they have now been married for 41 years. I guess it doesn't take the Ferrin men long to know what they want and go after it.

After giving Ryan his ring back, I had a thought that changed the trajectory of my life forever, "I deserve to be loved and happy. My girls deserve a good man in their life. And gosh darn it, he is worth the risk of another heart break." You guessed it! He gave me my ring back.

Allowing that fear to start settling in almost prevented me from making one of the best decisions I have ever made, allowing this man to love me and my girls the way we deserve and for us to love him back.

A little over a year after completing chemo, I married the man of my dreams. We are now going on 16 wonderful years of marriage. He has also adopted my girls who are now his girls.

I couldn't see in me what he saw in me because the lenses we were looking through were two totally different prescriptions. His eyes saw me for my heart. My eyes saw me for all the mistakes I had made.

The more I got to know Ryan, the more I respected his opinions of me, to the point that I eventually saw myself the way he did. I didn't know my worth all those years ago, but he helped me see it. He brought out in me what was already there. And over the years, I started to trust the mirror he was holding up.

That fear I had when I tried to break it off with him never came to fruition. I've learned a lot about love since then. One thing I know to be true is love really can heal a broken heart and love will never steer me wrong, if I allow it to be my north star. I've learned that my mistakes are not who I am, but experiences I had and that despite them, I am still worthy of love.

I refuse to let others tell us that luck is a part of our journey. Luck indicates that God's hand wasn't in the details of our beginning or that we didn't create the kind of marriage we now have, which was created through love and consistent work. Luck gets no credit for our marriage! We are blessed to have each other and the life we have created together.

Sweet sister, you are so worthy of love. If love is what you desire, it's yours. Trust in God's timing. It may not make sense to you or the world, and that's ok. You may find it in an unlikely person in an unlikely way. When love comes knocking, open your heart and welcome it in. Oh, how worthy of love you are.

"Beginnings are scary, endings are usually sad, but it's the middle that counts the most. You need to remember that when you find yourself at the beginning. Just give hope a chance to float up, and it will too."

-Hope Floats

Some struggles are
due to limiting beliefs
but once released,
so is the struggle.

#upstruggle

Chapter 4
The Forbidden

I grew up in a culture that taught if a mother could stay home and raise her kids, she should. How I interpreted this was, if I could stay home financially, I should. I can totally see the value in this teaching from my church, I really can. When my children were little, I was able to see the kid's excitement that it was my face they saw greeting them at the bus stop or greeting them at the front door. I loved that I got to be the first one to ask them how their day was.

I loved being able to witness those sweet babies run up to their dad every day when he got home from work and give him hugs and kisses. It was like watching a store be stormed when the doors opened on Black Friday. Now, the dog is the only one to greet him like that.

Still, staying home and having a desire to work caused conflict within myself. It's like something was calling me to work, but I was so worried that working outside the home would somehow screw my kids up. No, seriously. I know it's silly now, but I didn't know any better back then.

I didn't know the effects it would have on them because I was taught it was better for the kids and family as a whole if the mother stayed home. I didn't question it much.

I didn't want the kids coming home to an empty house. I didn't want them resenting me for always being gone. All they ever knew was that mom was always there when they got home from school. To some degree, I felt guilt for wanting to work. I had a husband who afforded me the opportunity to stay home, yet I knew other moms who had to work but wished they could stay home. There were women who wanted what I had, while I wanted what they had.

One day, I had this thought that changed my perspective on being a working mom. "You may be able to stay home financially, but you are not able to stay home mentally and emotionally." That was the game changer for me.

I wasn't looking for a full time job. Not that I think that is bad, because I don't. I just knew it wasn't what I wanted.

Just something that would get me out of the house and around grown-ups. I thought about what it was I wanted to do. What was on my heart? What was I passionate about? My answer – sick people. Having had been sick myself, it gave me a higher level of compassion for those dealing with an illness.

Immediately, I thought about working in a hospital. I did some research and learned about becoming a Certified Nursing Assistant. This wouldn't take long to get and got me out of the house immediately. This was something that if I wanted to take my education further in, I could.

Ryan was on board. He is always on board with whatever makes me happy. Off I went to my first class. I was in love. I had never been one to really love learning, but maybe it's because I had never taken time to learn about the things that interested me.

When I did my clinicals, I did them in a nursing home and quickly realized that was not where I wanted to be. I wanted to take more time with the people. I didn't want to rush my time with them. I even cried one time at clinicals. This man who was a bilateral amputee had been sitting in his own feces. Not only was he sitting in it, but he also had an open wound on his back side and was screaming as he was being cleaned up. My heart broke, and I knew I was not cut out for this kind of scene.

After getting certified, I did a little digging and learned about private home health care. This is where you go into someone's home and take care of them one on one. I liked this idea. I quickly found a job working for a man with ALS and worked with only ALS for about 5 years. I was able to work a few days a week like I wanted and make some pretty decent money too. Perks with working in private home health care! I made more money and could pick the days and hours I wanted to work.

Not only was I able to get out of the house, but I was able to do something I loved part time and still feel like I was home enough with my kids. I had found the perfect job for me and my family at that time in our life.

Believing that working would somehow screw my children up was my limiting belief I had to release. Maybe for you, your limiting belief that you are holding onto is thinking you don't deserve a promotion, so you don't go after it. Maybe it's that you think you are unlovable, so you push people away. Whatever it is, once you release it, you will also release the struggle accompanied with it.

We can't go sticking each other in boxes. We can't expect that what works for one mother will work for the next. There is not only one right way to raise a family. I know there is value in a mom who stays home and raises her kids. There is also value in working outside the home. For me, I was able to strike a really good balance for my family. My job allowed me to be home most days but also allowed me to fulfill a desire I had in my heart – working.

Working helped me build confidence in myself too. I felt happier because I was no longer stressed out all the time. Working allowed me to decompress and get a break from the kids. It even gave us extra spending cash to do fun things as a family. When I was home, I was home. When I was at work, I was at work. It truly made me a better mom and wife. As forbidden as it seemed, working was exactly what this mama needed!

Allow your struggles to level you up.

#upstruggle

Chapter 5
This-N-That Part 1

Hold that thought

Oh, sweet sister friend, this one was so hard for me to learn. But boy, oh boy, am I glad I finally learned it.

There was this one time, I mean there were plenty of times I should have held my thought but I'm going to share this one with you. There was this family that lived nearby, they had 4 children just like we did. They even had 2 girls and 2 boys close to all our children's ages. It's like each kid had their own friend. It was amazing! I enjoyed the wife. Ryan enjoyed the husband. We all got along, and I thought I had found a forever friend.

Now, I don't recall all the details, but one of my daughters had a falling out with one of their daughters. At first, I didn't think it would cause a huge issue. I figured the girls would make up and it would blow by. How wrong I was.

It got to the point that it affected our friendship because that girl pulled her mom into it, and then the mom started to treat me differently. You know, the whole ignoring me, no longer inviting us over, hurtful words getting back to me that were said about my daughter or us as parents, stuff like that.

For some reason, this blew up so dang big. It was so toxic that church leaders got involved. It was affecting the whole young woman's youth program at our church. Even other adults were dragged into it. My mind was blown. This was the kind of drama that took place with other people and certainly something I swore would never be on my front doorstep. Like ever.

Anyway, trying to resolve the issue took place through text because the mom was so hard to talk to in person. Hard as in she made it difficult by ignoring me and clearly not wanting to talk to me.

Long story short, I found myself texting the mom and Ryan at the same time. We were trying to resolve the issue that started off with our girls but now had our entire church involved. Talk about embarrassing.

I can't remember what all was said back and forth between Ryan and this lady, but I do remember feeling really frustrated that it wasn't going anywhere positive. This was said in a text that was meant for Ryan, "Screw them!" I mean, it also said something along the lines of I'm done, this isn't going anywhere. But it definitely said, "Screw them!" That I will never forget because I ended up sending that text to the mom instead of Ryan! Oh my gosh! Smack hand to forehand and then do it again moment.

I was so embarrassed. I quickly told Ryan what I had done. There was no taking it back. I knew at this point, there definitely was no chance at resolving the issue. That ended up being the case.

This experience taught me a few lessons. In no specific order. Ok, besides maybe number 1.

1. Oh my gosh, always double check and make sure your text message is going to the right person. Especially those risqué pictures you send your husband from time to time. Triple check those, sister! Please, don't act like you don't do that too.

2. Hold that thought and calm down before releasing it. Most often than not, once you are calm, your thoughts will be totally different. Like much nicer and clearer.

3. Some people come into your life for a reason, season, or a lifetime. She was clearly the first 2. I learned a lot from this and my friendship with her.

4. What you focus on is what you get more of. I could have easily ignored it all, but I didn't. Mainly because I was so hurt

by the things being said, and I felt like it was a friendship worth trying to save. I allowed myself to put way too much focus on it.

5. I cannot control what others say or do, but I can always control how I react to what they say or do.

I always go back to this one experience when I find myself wanting to say something unkind. No, this doesn't mean we can't be direct and honest. I respect people who are direct and honest. But I believe no one should ever use the excuse, "I'm just direct and honest" as an excuse to be rude. #growthtookplace

Use the other door

There's something I've noticed at my gym, about 80% of the people who walk through the gym doors use the door that is harder to open. It's not that they don't know this door has more resistance than the one right next to it. It's labeled, and you have to push a button so it will open for you. Yet, they still choose the door that makes them struggle. Sometimes I even get a good chuckle out of watching them do this. Shhhh......

Every time I see someone use this door, I wonder why, when the other door leads to the exact same place but has far less resistance.

Not only do they do this once, but they do it with the second set of doors.

How often do you choose the door with more resistance in life?

How often do you make relationships more complicated than they need to be?

How often do you make life harder on yourself than it needs to be?

There are multiple doors that lead to the same place in life, yet so many of us choose the door that gives the most resistance. Why?

I think sometimes people choose the door with more resistance for a few reasons. Reasons like I did for many years.

I thought life was meant to be hard. And if it's not, I must have been doing something wrong. I must not be trying hard enough. I must not be growing enough. Although growth will require discomfort, life is NOT meant to be like that 100% of the time. I just assumed life was supposed to be hard to the point that when things were going well, I would tell myself, "Enjoy it, because this won't last."

For many years, I made choices that caused more resistance in my life than needed because that's what I thought I deserved. I thought I didn't deserve better. So, in a subconscious way, I would sabotage myself. Looking for the door that is harder to open.

I lived on autopilot and wasn't thinking about the actions I was taking. Just letting life take me where it wanted instead of choosing where I wanted to go. I was part of that 80% using the door with more resistance until one day I realized what I was doing and stopped.

I'm a huge believer that life is what we choose it to be. It's a manifestation of a whole lot of choices, thoughts, and beliefs.

Now don't get me wrong, God has a lot of say too. And we know we can't control other people's actions which can affect our lives. But we do have total control over ourselves, our reactions, our beliefs, and our choices.

Know this, God doesn't want your life to be hard. And other times, those trials we experience, we bring upon ourselves because of the door we choose to use. When we think life is supposed to be hard, we choose the door with far more resistance, when literally, right next to it is a door that leads to the exact same place but has less resistance.

Choose your door, my friend! And choose it wisely.

Self-talk

I won't lie, I struggled with negative self-talk. I struggled with always comparing myself to others. I struggled with having my photo taken. I struggled with being complimented.

I couldn't see my own worth or strengths. Because I allowed myself to be blinded by my weaknesses.

I thought I was being "humble". Humble my butt. That's not humble.

I realized I couldn't love others the way they deserved until I first loved myself. I couldn't treat others the way they deserved until I treated myself better.

You know, life is a journey. It's about growth. It's about loving who we are and appreciating ourselves while we work on becoming a bit better.

We have to be careful not to fall into the trap of, "I am perfect the way I am so no need for improvement."

And we have to be careful of falling into the trap of, "I am not enough, and therefore I must work like a crazy person to become better."

I've done both and I can promise you, neither brought me joy!

I believe we can find a happy balance. Yes, we do need to work on ourselves. The moment we think we are perfect is the moment we start moving backwards.

And the moment we think we aren't enough is the moment we lose our joy!

I've played both games. And each time, I lost. These are games that no one ever wins!!

Check yourself out in the mirror...no, I didn't say start picking yourself apart. Knock it off!!

Truly look at yourself. What are you good at? What character strengths do you possess? What are those things people always compliment you about? What do you like about your body?

I said...what...do...you...like!? Focus on these things. Be kind to yourself.

Sister, stop beating yourself up! Would you ever allow a friend to talk to you the way you talk to yourself sometimes?! Absolutely not.

If your child could hear your self-talk, would you be ok with it?! Would you ever talk to your child the way you sometimes talk to yourself? Absolutely not.

When we know our worth, we will stop doing things that are harmful to our souls.

It's a process. I won't lie! Nothing changes overnight. But aren't you with it?! Isn't your child worth having a happy mother?!

Most of the time, kids grow up to be like their parents. Are you ok with that?

Everyone struggles, some just do it better.

#upstruggle

Chapter 6
Am I making the right choice?

Am I making the right choice? What if this is the wrong decision? What if I am making the biggest mistake of my life? What if this is a waste of my time? What if it doesn't work out?

Does any of that sound familiar? Yup, they're things I have said to myself too. I get it. Maybe you have found yourself saying this about a job, relationship, move, what school to attend, who to marry, what degree to get, etc.

But here's a question I have for you. How will you ever really know if it was the right or wrong choice to begin with? Like is some fairy god mother going to come to you and tell you that you made the right or wrong choice? If so, can you send her my way?

Let's say you make a decision and it does work out; who's to say that the other one wouldn't have been better for you? How would you even know that the other one wouldn't have been better for you? I don't say this to freak you out or make you second guess your decision. But to prove a point.

I mean, I do believe that sometimes we will have a very peaceful feeling about a certain decision we are making but not always. At least that's been my experience.

Because sometimes it's our own limiting beliefs that can create tension within us. That doesn't mean that what we want is wrong. It just means that our mindset needs to shift so that we don't feel so uneasy about doing the thing we want to do.

Kind of like when I wanted to work. I had to release the limiting belief that working meant I would screw my kids up or miss out on blessings. Once I released that limiting belief, I was able to have peace with that decision. A decision that has brought nothing but happiness and joy to not just my life but my family's life.

I believe when we work a decision out in our minds and come up with two good options, and take it to God, often times he will leave it up to us to choose. I can't tell you how many times I've heard, "Neither choice is wrong, you choose."

I also used to think that if I get the outcome I wanted, it was the right choice, but that if I didn't get the outcome I wanted, then it was the wrong choice.

I disagree with that way of thinking now. How do you know that just because you didn't get the outcome you wanted; it means it was the wrong choice?

Sometimes we need to experience things to go to the next level. Sometimes we aren't ready for the outcome we want when we want it. And maybe, just maybe, we need to fail a lot more, so we are ready to receive the outcome we want when it comes our way.

Back in 2016, I was 110% inspired to become a Beachbody coach. I'm talking, it felt so right in my soul. A Beachbody coach is a virtual health coach that helps other people get healthy. My job was to become a better version of myself and also help other ladies do the same. I ran monthly online fitness groups helping women (and a few men too) lose weight but also helped them work on their mindset.

Because something I know, being overweight is never really about the weight to begin with, but a deeper issue, and the way that issue manifests itself is through being overweight. This is where working on the mind helps. Because when we learn to shed limiting beliefs, we will begin to shed the pounds, literally and figuratively.

As I would talk to these ladies, this became very evident to me. I worked with ladies who had low self-esteem, lacked confidence, were timid, didn't believe in themselves, and all the things we women experience at some point in our lives.

As I started to help them work on their mindset, they began making lifestyle changes because that's the evolution of feeling better about who you are and knowing what you deserve.

I knew nothing about online coaching. Thankfully, I signed up with a successful coach who had already been doing it for a few years and was willing to guide me through it all.

I didn't have an online presence. I didn't know how to set up a group on Facebook. I mean, there was a lot I didn't know. I had to learn everything. And it's safe to say that in the beginning, I sucked.

But the more I did it, the better I got. I was helping women all over the country get fit mentally and physically.

I was meeting new people online. I was getting healthy myself. I was moving my business along. I was making a presence for myself on social media. I earned a trip with my Coach to attend the High Performance academy by Brendon Burchard who is the world's leading high performance coach, a New York Times bestselling author, and has been on stage with Rachel Hollis.

I earned a team retreat with the top coaches on our team, which was paid for by my coach.

Often times, I would receive messages from people I was connected with on social media, telling me how much I had helped change their lives or helped them through a tough time. That alone would make my day! I was happy that I was able to do that for someone else by doing this online coaching business.

I mean, I felt like this was "it." You know what I mean? Like, this was the thing I was meant to do outside of being a wife and a mother.

Not long after all this, I started to feel like this was not what I was meant to do for the rest of my life. This was not the thing I was being prepared for. But wait a minute, I felt it impressed upon me that I should do this and that it was the right choice to move forward with, so why isn't it working out the way I thought it would? Why am I having these feelings?

The decision to no longer be a health coach was a really tough choice for me to make. It didn't make sense to me. I didn't understand why I felt God led me down this path only for it to not work out the way I had envisioned. It seemed cruel, and I was frustrated.

Little did I know that at that time, I was meant to choose that path in my life. But it was merely a steppingstone to where I would be going.

I would not be sitting here writing this book if it weren't for being a coach. Part of being a coach meant I had to be present on social media and make posts. Not just any posts. Posts that added value to the readers. Posts that were from the heart. Posts that left me exposed to criticism. I had to learn how to be vulnerable and write in a way that others could connect to. Because hiding and not being real meant not connecting with anyone. Connection was vital in building that business.

Adding value on social media and talking about the hard things at the same time took some practice for sure!

Hands down, it's where I learned how to write. Because this girl has no degree or any formal training that taught her how. I have now been writing consistently for 4 years.

I've even been teased about how long my posts are. Thank goodness they were, because I have been able to go back to those posts and use some of the content for this book.

At first, I sucked hard core at writing. Not saying I'm the best now but certainly much better. At first, I was worried about what others would think or say about me. I mean, it was hard to expose myself to people on the internet. I can't tell you how many times I would post and ghost. Because I was too afraid of what people might comment on it.

It helped me build up the confidence to share my story and journey openly. To not get so caught up on worrying about what others might say or think about me.

Just because the coaching thing didn't work out the way I envisioned, didn't make it the wrong choice or mean it didn't work out just how it was supposed to. Without it, I wouldn't be where I am today. So much goodness has come out of me making that decision. It served its purpose in my life. It was the exact steppingstone I needed.

Take divorce for example. A marriage is never a waste of time just because it didn't work out. Just because it didn't work out doesn't mean it was a wrong decision either. Did you have children together? You wouldn't have those babies if you didn't marry him. Did you learn what you will and won't put up with now? Did you also grow as an individual during that time? Did you meet your best friend which would have never happened if your husband didn't get that job promotion that took you across the country?

When we are in it, we can't always see why it happens the way it does, but looking back, we can always see how one path we chose that didn't work out how we thought it would, actually worked out exactly how it was supposed to.

You see, it's all about how you choose to look at it. Does that really sound like the wrong decision to you? Does that sound like a mistake or a waste of time? I don't think so.

struggles don't make
you weak, they
make you human.

#upstruggle

Chapter 7

Just stay

"Life is a game, play it. Life is too precious, do not destroy it."

-Mother Teresa

I don't often talk about my dating years since I've been happily married for almost 16 years, and honestly, it feels weird.

But I'm going to because I feel impressed to share this one story.

I was about 15 when I had the worst break up ever. Not that the breakup itself was bad or terrible. The heartbreak from it was.

I had been dating this guy who was a really good guy. He treated me good. He was respectful to me. He was sweet and kind. He was the kind of guy any mom would be thrilled to have their daughter dating.

We dated for what seemed like forever. When you are that young, dating for over a year is a really long time.

As a teen, it's true that you can't always see past your own nose. I saw everything up close, never taking a step back to see the full picture.

He broke up with me, and because I didn't have the maturity needed to handle that kind of pain, I decided in order to make it go away, I would swallow an entire bottle of Tylenol.

Or at least whatever was in the bottle. I don't know how many. I didn't count. I just took.

After I did that and I started to physically feel sick, I realized how stupid it was. I called my mom to tell her what I had just done.

By the time my mom and a family friend arrived, I was curled up in a ball slowing drifting in and out. They did whatever they could to keep me awake. I know a blessing (a blessing is like saying a prayer over someone that is inspired from God) was administered to me.

As I was being loaded up into the ambulance, one of the EMT's said to my mom, "Why would she do this?! She's such a pretty girl."

Out of that entire experience, that is the one thing that has always stayed with me and is crystal clear.

Because as soon as he said that, I wanted to vomit. Like forget sticking the tube down my nose and pumping some ugly black stuff down it, I will happily vomit for you.

Like somehow because I have a pretty face, I'm not allowed to struggle. I'm not allowed to experience pain. I'm not allowed to do stupid things. I'm not allowed to get dumped. My life is supposed to go a certain way.

Like somehow a nice face gives anyone a free pass in life from experiencing struggles.

Out of it all, the hospital stay, the stomach pumping, the friends coming to visit, the therapist, all of it, that is what I remember so vividly.

I think, to some degree, we all say this to each other in one way or another. I've been so guilty of it myself.

Why is she so unhappy, she has a wonderful husband!

Why would she yell at her kids, she has the best kids ever!

Why would she quit her job, she has the best job ever!

Why is she going through bankruptcy, she makes plenty of money!

Why is she having a panic attack, she seems to have it all together!

Why would she think no one likes her, she is loved by everyone!

Why would she do something so stupid, she had everything going for her!

Why is she so negative, she grew up in such a positive home!

Like somehow only certain people are allowed to struggle. Only certain faces can struggle. Only people with certain jobs, bank accounts, or relationships are allowed to struggle.

Show me one person who says they have never had struggles in their life, and I will show you a huge liar with some massive issues needing to be worked through.

Yes, it's true this one was self-induced.

True, some people struggle more than others. And yes, I believe sometimes, those people struggle more because of their own choices. But regardless, no one is exempt. No one.

And remember, nothing in life is ever so bad that it won't get better with some pure grit. Nothing in this life is ever worth taking your own life and causing even more pain.

Instead of thinking suicide is the best option, learn from and understand the purpose of your struggles. Put your ego and pride aside so you can find the lessons from it. Reach out for help. Talk to someone. Find a good therapist.

It wasn't until I came to the understanding that I wasn't the only one who had struggles, some just hid theirs really well, that I was no longer ashamed of mine.

I started to look at struggles as opportunities to grow. Opportunities to learn. Opportunities to help others get through what I went through. Opportunities to show courage and strength. Just flat out opportunities!

I promise, things do get better if you begin to take action. And making a mental shift and flipping the script to serve you really helps too!

You are not alone. No, I may not understand your exact struggle, and you may not understand mine. But you and I know struggle. We know pain. I know that tunnel may seem so dark and never ending, but if you keep putting one foot in front of the other, eventually you will see the light.

Trust your struggles. Trust they are feedback. They are there to help you grow. Trust in a loving God who wants to see you conquer them.

If life feels like one big struggle, sister, that is not what life is meant to feel like. That is feedback that something has to shift within yourself. Yes, you will have seasons of struggle, but life itself isn't meant to feel like one big struggle.

Stay in the game! Learn from your struggle so you can play the game better.

For help, call The National Suicide Prevention Lifeline. They are available 24 hours a day. 1-800-273-8255

Or visit their website at www.suicidepreventionlifeline.org for more details or to chat with someone online.

Asking for help does not make you weak. Asking for help takes a certain level of strength, which is why it's so hard to do. Be strong.

struggle is not a
nasty word, stop
making it one.

#upstruggle

Chapter 8
Therapy #noshame

What you feed your mind matters. If we don't intentionally fill our minds with good things, the adversary is more than happy to fill it with crap worthy things. I didn't understand the power of reading until four years ago. And when I say it has changed my life, that is an understatement.

How often do you eat? 3, 4, 5, 6, times a day? Sounds about right, huh? A little different person to person.

We feed our bodies several times a day to keep it going. If we stop eating, we starve. We feel like crap. We have hunger pains. We lose an unhealthy amount of weight. Nothing good comes from starving ourselves.

No one in their right mind says, "I think I will just stop eating because I know I will feel so much better if I do." No one says that! If anything, some of us overeat. Hey, I'm so guilty of that too. #notjudging

We know from infancy that we need to eat, or we feel bad. We understand this concept. So naturally, we eat when we are hungry. Our bodies are really good at telling us when we need to eat.

But, what about our minds? Our minds are starving for good food too. As often as we feed our body, we should feed our minds. Yes. That means several times a day. No, I'm not joking!

Just like the quality of food we feed our body matters, so does the quality of food we feed our minds. When we eat junk food, we feel bad. When we consume junk magazines, movies, music, or books, we feel bad too.

A friend sent me a quote the other day that said, "You are not born a winner. You are not born a loser. You are born a chooser."

What floats around in your mind is a choice. It's like the one thing we do have control over. What and how we choose to think. Those first thoughts, the ones that might be a little crazy, we all have them. It's what you do with them that you are accountable for. Dwelling on them or chalking them up to silly thoughts that must go, is on you. I've learned that in order to live a high-quality life, I must take care of my mind.

How you feed your mind may look different from how I do. What matters is that you feed it. The power is in your hands. Our lives are a manifestation of the quality of our thoughts.

So why neglect the mind? Our minds are starving for good nutrition. Take time to feed yours daily.

Feeding our minds is not a one and done kind of thing. Remember, they need to eat as often as our bodies. For some of us, maybe more. Just depends on how long it's been starving and how ingrained the unhealthy thinking is.

So next time you look at someone and wonder why they are so positive and happy. No, they were not just born that way or got lucky, or just grew up in the right family. They choose it and so can you. You are worth it! And by golly, the people who have to be around us 24/7 are worth it too, huh?

I am a huge advocate for "self-help" books, or as we readers like to call them, personal development books. After no longer being an online health and fitness coach, personal development was still something I continued to do. It had changed my life so much there was no way I was going to give it up just because I was no longer a coach. I felt in my soul this was something being a coach was meant to bring into my life.

Here's how I look at it. People go to therapy when they have an issue, yes?

They pay someone else to help them figure out how to get through a problem, how to deal with a difficult loved one, or whatever their issue is. But regardless of that issue, they are seeking a solution to a problem. They are seeking help from another source.

And no one bats an eye or says, "You really don't need that. You have the scriptures, prayer, and the spirit to guide you out of whatever your problem is!" No freaking way have I ever heard that before. If anything, I hear, "Don't be ashamed to go. Seek professional help!"

And I would agree! Seek professional help if you need to, no shame in that!

I think what a lot of people fail to understand about "self-help" books is it's actually just another form of therapy.

At least for me and everyone I know who read the books. These books help explain the issue, how they got through it, different ways of thinking, and offer solutions. Sounds like a form of therapy to me! Sometimes the scriptures make even more sense after I've read a book.

I read books based on a few reasons:

1. What am I currently struggling with that I would like to better understand so I can be better at it? Isn't that why people go to therapy?

2. What am I interested in learning more about? Sounds pretty educational to me.

3. What is a loved one struggling with that I want to better understand? Sounds like a pretty good reason to read a "self-help" book.

I believe that God has gifted people with the ability to reach into the minds of others to help them see things in a way that serves them. This gift wasn't just for those of old. This is a modern day gift too.

No, I do not believe that if someone is suffering or struggling that if they just read their scriptures, pray, have faith, all will be well.

That makes me laugh. So, if you are suffering and do all those things and nothing helps, just sit in your suffering and have faith. Like what? No way, sister! Keep searching.

I do believe we need to figure out what works for each one of us as an individual and stop trying to put people in a box. Like it's this one way and it's the only way to do it. That is silly.

Maybe reading the scriptures is all you need. Maybe I just haven't learned how to get them to help me figure out every aspect of life.

But, thankfully, I have figured out what to couple them with to help me continue progressing in this life. Coupling the scriptures with personal development books has been a recipe for massive growth in my life. They keep me moving forward.

Not to mention that the leaders in my church quote these books during their talks. Heck, some even write these books. Must be something to them, huh?

I keep a running list of all the books I've read or listened to. You can head over to my website at TraceyFerrin.com and download the list for free.

Struggles are like reps. The more you do, the stronger you become.

#upstruggle

Chapter 9
It's there for a reason

One day, about 8 years ago, a friend from church invited me to go workout at her gym, and when she said I could bring my kids and put them in daycare, I was all over that! I fell in love with this gym right away. This was a really nice gym, and I wanted to join, so I convinced my husband to let me.

At that time in our life, the gym membership was really out of our budget, and the 20min drive would also add to our gas bill. You know, that time in your marriage where you have to make your tank last so many days or else. The gym I wanted to join was like a county club. It wasn't your 20 bucks a month kind of gym.

How was I going to make this work? When we really want something, we always find a way to make it work, right? I told Ryan I would cut back on eating out and my friend and I would take turns driving to the gym. Yes, I ate out that much. No, I'm not proud to admit that. Yes, I still eat out that much.

I was hooked! Everything I did for the day revolved around me getting to the gym to workout. Doctor appointments, play dates, everything revolved around my dedication to my workouts. I even packed our lunches for the day because remember, I was eating out less so I could afford the membership.

I quickly realized that I loved the group fitness classes. I was taking strength training and cycle classes. Oh, and some mat Pilates as well. I had my favorite instructors and never missed a class. And if there was a sub one day, oh, how I was not happy about it. Like what could possibly be more important than teaching their class? Surely, instructors don't have a life outside teaching...

I went from being a sideline mom to playing in the game. I went from telling my kids I didn't have energy to play with them to the point of them asking me if we could stop playing because they were exhausted.

This new lifestyle made me feel so good that I had the crazy idea to become a group fitness instructor. I wanted every woman to feel as good as working out made me feel, and I wanted to impact their lives like these instructors had mine. I still remember all their names. James was my spin instructor. Becky was my Pilates instructor. Sherah was my strength training instructor.

The thought that I could one day teach classes and change lives like mine had been, festered inside me. I felt strongly that I needed to do this. I ordered my materials and couldn't wait to dive in and start studying. When the books arrived, I was in complete shock. It was talking about the heart, lunges, muscles, bones, diet, and so much more. I mean, it had words I couldn't even spell much less pronounce.

I was like, I'm not trying to be a nurse, I just want to teach some classes. It intimidated me, and I questioned if I would even be able to pass the test. You want to know what I did with the books? I let them collect dust for a good year before I had the courage to pick them back up and go all in. It took me close to another year to study all the material and feel confident that I had prepared as much as I possibly could.

I scheduled my test, then prayed and fasted that I would pass. I've never been a good test taker, so I was diligent in my studies but knew I needed a little extra help from above.

I'm happy to announce, I did pass the test, and on the first try! I was so excited and couldn't wait to start teaching. I even started teaching at the same club I was a member of. This was very much so one of those full circle moments for me.

It was a dream come true because this gym doesn't just take any instructor. You have to audition to work there, and you have to have 1 year of teaching under your belt. I mean, by no means was I at the level of the more seasoned instructors. But I knew with practice, I could get there.

After working there for a year, I was asked to be one of their ELI (Exclusive Lifetime Instructor) instructors. Being an ELI comes with some perks.

Perks like having really good health, vision, and dental insurance. We now save over a thousand dollars each month just by removing the kids and I off Ryan's insurance and putting them on mine. Ryan and I got Invisalign. We put 2 kids through braces and have our last one in. All with no out of pocket cost. Yup, that's how good the insurance is.

These are things our family might have missed out on had I let fear hold me back from doing what was in my heart. Being an instructor even helped prepare me for public speaking. I was already used to using a mic, standing on stage, and talking in front of a group of people. Just in a slightly different way, of course! Before I started public speaking, I had been teaching for almost 5 years. That's 5 years of practicing public speaking. Which I would have missed out on had I not followed my heart.

Getting certified turned me into a believer that with hard work, I could accomplish anything and that when something is placed on my heart, it's for a reason.

Coming to the point I am at today was not easy, but I wouldn't be here had I given up on something I really wanted and knew deep down, I was supposed to do. God places things in our hearts not to torture us but to guide us. He knows we can do hard things. Never let the size of the climb scare you from even starting.

No, becoming a fitness instructor may not be for you, or maybe it is, I don't know. But doing things that challenge you and make you feel good about yourself is. Never forget, you are setting the example for your children, especially your daughters. How can you ever tell them to go after their dreams and that they are capable of accomplishing anything if you didn't show them how? How can you teach them to listen to what's in their heart if you don't listen to what's in yours?

What is in your heart that you are not honoring because the climb seems too big? Commit today to start working towards that thing. Small steps still move the needle forward. Sister, the time will pass anyway. So why not do the thing that is on your heart?

Let what's on your heart guide you. As scary as it can be, that's why it's there. I promise it will never lead you astray.

Don't be the cause
of someone else's
struggle. Be the
light they need and
the reason they get
through it.

#upstruggle

Chapter 10
This-N-That Part 2

Consider the source

At one point in my life, I had someone who would tell me everything someone else would say about me. I wouldn't feed into the conversations, and I think this person started wondering why it wasn't ruffling my feathers and why I wasn't getting mad over it. I finally spoke up and said, "I'm considering the (the source talked about everyone and liked to point their finger at everyone) source. I don't too much care for what they are saying as much as I care that you would keep repeating what they say."

If someone has something hurtful to say about someone else, please tell me the purpose of running to that person and repeating it? A lot of the time, it just causes drama and hurts feelings. Not sure how that is helpful.

Yes, I get sometimes it may be necessary, but truth be told, I can't really think of too many times where it was.

It's not our job to make sure everyone likes us. It is however our job to be authentic in who we are. Yes, it is a human desire to want people to like us, but who likes us matters more than having everyone like us.

If someone doesn't like you, does it really matter? Does it affect your life? If yes, it's time for a sit down with that person. But release the need to be liked by everyone. You will always be too much for some, not enough for others, and just right for the people who want and need you in their lives.

Where you put your energy matters. Time is not something we can get back. But it is something we often waste.

Here are two questions that help me.

1. Did I do something to that person that would cause them to not like me? If so, sincerely ask for forgiveness. What happens past that is on them.

2. Is there truth to what they are saying? Yes? Work on your ish. No? Move on.

Consider the source. Bless and release.

What I mean is this. Does this person not like anyone? Does this person talk about everyone? Does this person hold high regards in your life? No? Then don't worry. Them not liking you is not your problem, it's theirs. It's their own insecurities surfacing. That is none of your business, sweet friend.

Oprah style

Ever felt like you lost a part of who you are because all you ever say is yes to everyone?

Hey, I get it! That was me many years ago. Until I discovered the word NO.

When I first started telling people no, it was a little uncomfortable. But the more I said it, the more natural it became.

Like Oprah style...you get a no, and you get a no, you all get a no!!!

I usually use the word no when someone asks me to do something last minute. Yes, I'm a planner. I believe everyone should be to some extent.

Now your last-minute definition and my last-minute definition could be two totally different definitions, and that's ok!

My definition of last-minute is when someone asks me to do something and it encroaches on my schedule, meaning I would have to change my plans to accommodate them. They get a no.

Or, if what they ask of me makes me feel rushed. Feeling rushed creates anxiety, and I don't like that feeling. They get a no.

I refuse to feel rushed or anxious because other people don't know how to plan in advance.

And I'm not talking about an emergency where a friend or family member needs help or something. Of course, we should help out in those cases. That's when I'm willing to rearrange my schedule.

I'm talking more about day to day things that people wait till the last minute to drop in our lap. Things that they could have easily put forth a little effort to plan. But because they operate in chaos or don't care about our time, they ask last minute.

I believe using the word no sets boundaries. I've experienced this here lately, and that's why it's been on my mind. Let me tell you something I know, if we are constantly allowing people to drop last minute things on our plate, they will continue to do that. People do what we allow them to.

And when you tell someone no, don't apologize for it. Simply tell them you can't, but if you had more notice, you would have loved to. Kindly let them know how much notice you would need for something they are asking you to do.

The day I decided to set boundaries with my time and last-minute things was the day I started to take back control of my life. If you are not telling people no, you are not truly in charge of your own life. Get comfortable telling people no.

This is your time and your life.

When quitting is necessary

Hear me out, I know what you're thinking, quitting is not a good habit to have. There is a difference between quitting and giving up.

Giving up is not an option because you are struggling, and you want the struggle to be over with. Because you know if you give up, that tension you feel will subside. It's not an option because something is hard. It's not an option because a goal is taking longer than you thought. It's not an option because you are not good at something right away. That comes with time. That's when we don't give up.

So, when is it okay to quit?

I've learned it's ok to quit when priorities change. It's ok to quit if you realize something is just not for you.

Do quit if better opportunities arise. Like a better job opportunity. You would have to be crazy to turn down that just because you didn't want to "quit." Like my chemo, I had to quit because I knew it was killing me. It was no longer serving me but hurting me.

Redirecting your focus and energy is ok!

Often times we have to try something out to know whether we like it or not, and if we don't, it's ok to quit. If you are anything like me, you have to dabble in many things to see what it is you really do enjoy. We are forever changing and evolving humans, that means what we like may change too. #multipassionate

I mean, would you keep painting, doing pottery, photography, just because you invested in it but realize you hate it? No way!! Doesn't make sense. At this point, you are taking from the things that are truly important to you and holding yourselves back from being successful in the aspects you truly want to be successful in.

This is when it's time to quit, when it is no longer for you but against you.

If you work for a company where you don't believe in their values and you don't believe in the direction they're going, are you really going to stay with them? No way!! I mean, maybe long enough so you can find a new job. But you want to align yourself with a company you can support and feel confident working for. Right? Of course.

You see, I've learned that there are times when it's absolutely necessary to quit, but I've also learned that I can't give up just because things are hard.

I've learned that even when I quit, so much growth still takes place. So, was it pointless? Nope! I learned and moved on. I've taken those things and applied them to other aspects of life. Sounds like a win to me!

I'm so guilty of it too, sometimes I get my hands in so many different things that I spread myself thin, and I realize, it is time to sit down and reprioritize what's truly important to me. Somethings may need to go on the back burner and somethings I may need to let go of altogether.

Don't waste time worrying about what others will think by you quitting. Because sometimes quitting is absolutely necessary in order to move forward.

Never forget, saying no to one thing opens up space in your life to say yes to things that truly matter to you. To the things of far better worth.

Know when quitting serves you and when it doesn't.

There is a cost to personal growth, often times that cost will come in the form of a struggle.

#upstruggle

Chapter 11

The white coats

"You already have 3; you should be grateful for them and not have anymore."

"You should consider tying your tubes."

"If you get pregnant again, it could kill you. I recommend you not have any more babies."

That's what the doctors told me. One was an OBGYN, and the other was my Cardiologist.

Ryan and I knew we wanted a fourth child. But at that time, I was having health issues.

I had what was called a complete molar pregnancy. Where your body thinks it's pregnant and acts like it is but really isn't. It's just a mass growing inside your uterus.

We had to remove it by doing a D&C. My gynecological oncologist told me she usually has people do chemo for this kind of thing just to be sure it doesn't come back and or turn into cancer. But with my history and everything I had already gone through, she said would not make me do it and that she would make sure she scrapped me really good when removing the mass.

She also wanted to monitor me for an entire year after my D&C and told me I could absolutely positively not get pregnant during this time. I agreed.

I did blood work each week to make sure my HCG level was steadily dropping. Once it dropped to normal, I moved to monthly blood work to make sure my HCG stayed normal and didn't rise. A molar pregnancy spikes it crazy high. Like through the roof! Which is why your body thinks it's pregnant but also why this "pregnancy" usually feels different.

She told me that if my numbers didn't drop just once...just once, I would have to do chemo.

Imagine those phone calls. I had to do blood work and wait for the call for them to tell me if I was ok or if it was time to do chemo.

Finally, a year went by, and my levels had stayed normal for several months, so she cleared me to get pregnant. We started trying for another child. We got pregnant, then I had a miscarriage.

During this time, I also had cardiomyopathy. Well, that's what my cardiologist told me anyway. He thought it was caused from all the chemo I did a few years before.

My cardiologist told me I shouldn't have any more kids because the pregnancy could put too much stress on my heart.

I told him I appreciated his advice, but the final decision was between my husband and me.

I told Ryan that I knew without a doubt that a fourth baby was meant to come to our family. I felt to my core that having another baby would not kill me. I wasn't sure if it would do more damage to my heart, but that was a risk I was willing to take to bring that fourth child to our family. Did I think I was pushing the envelope with this one? Yeah! Could I actually go against doctor's advice not once but twice and have 2 good outcomes? Sure could!

We got pregnant! My cardiologist said he wanted to monitor me very closely during it, and I agreed to it.

My heart stayed the same till the end of my pregnancy when they performed my last echocardiogram. I was told my heart looked like it actually improved a little......WHILE BEING PREGNANT! What?!

What I failed to mention was that I had been through a handful of cardiologists already. All telling me that I had this heart problem. All trying to place limitations on me. And this whole time, something felt off with it all. I couldn't place my finger on it, but I knew something was off.

I remember one time Ryan asked me if I kept going through doctors because I didn't like what they were telling me. There was some truth to that but not in how he asked the question. He asked it in a way that conveyed me being in denial. It was about what they were saying and how it didn't feel right in my heart. To the point that I actually took myself off the meds my doctor had me on because every time I would take the pill, I felt like I was doing something wrong. I felt like I was harming my body, not helping it. I physically couldn't bring myself to taking those small little white pills any longer. Coreg anyone?

In 2012, I went to MDACC for a checkup. In this checkup, not only did they do blood work, take x-rays, do a PET scan, but they also did a MUGA (multiple-gated acquisition) scan. Now, a MUGA scan is superior to an echocardiogram. Did you know that? I sure didn't. A MUGA scan is specifically for measuring the ejection fraction (EF) of your heart.

When I went in to receive all my test results and talk to my oncologist, I asked him how my heart was. He told me fine. I let him know that it wasn't. That actually, I had cardiomyopathy. He told me I didn't and showed me the results. I was in shock. So many emotions surfaced, especially feeling upset and confused. Maybe my heart condition cleared up? Maybe they didn't care enough to run the tests needed and just wanted my money, yes, I went there.

I asked for a report of the scan so I could send it to my cardiologist, but not until after I asked my cardiologist to send me documentation saying I had cardiomyopathy. Once he did that, then I sent him the document from MDACC saying that in fact, I did not have a heart condition like he said.

You see, I was diagnosed with this condition when I was pregnant with our third child. That was all the way back in 2004. For 8 years, I was told I had a heart condition.

When I sent that 2012 scan to my doctor, you want to know what his response was? "A MUGA scan is superior to an echocardiogram. Echocardiograms have room for error."

Room for error! Are you kidding me! An EF of 36% (echocardiogram) and an EF of 56% (MUGA scan) is a lot of error! That error caused me to be on meds I didn't need. That error caused doctors to tell me to not have any more kids because it could kill me. And if a MUGA scan is far more superior, why wasn't that ran by my cardiologist? Why didn't he ask me if I had ever done one before? Why didn't he pull my records from MDACC to see what they said about my heart and what test they ran? Why weren't any extra steps taken?

As upset as I was, I just had to let it go. I could see where I was headed with all those questions and the feelings that I felt. I knew going down that rabbit hole was not going to lead me anywhere good. What could I actually do about it anyway? There is no going back and changing it. It had happened, that was a fact. And what I did moving forward and how I felt was now on me. I chose to do what made me feel better, I decided to let it go and move on. But trust me when I tell you, I learned from it.

Oh sister, I'm not done.

My husband applied for an increase of life insurance on me.

Like the kind that will pay for far more than just my funeral expenses when I die. Having had so many health issues, getting insurance wasn't cheap. But since I was more than 10 years out from cancer, we were ready to bump it up. We didn't know what having had a heart condition would do, but now that we knew I no longer had it, maybe they would clear me and give us a good rate.

As I was digging for documents to submit to the insurance company, I discovered a document from a 2005 scan. That scan said my heart was healthy (54% EF) too. I couldn't believe my eyes! Forget thinking that maybe I reversed my heart condition through health and fitness along the way, I was now convinced I never had cardiomyopathy to begin with.

Again, I was mad and confused. And all those feelings from the first time came flooding back. Crazy, right? But I did have to take some responsibility here. No, I'm not a doctor, but I do believe in being proactive in my own health, and I should have done more research. I put too much trust into the healthcare industry. That was on me. I knew something was off, and I knew I didn't feel right taking those meds. Somehow, I too had overlooked the 2005 scan results.

The life insurance agent took MD Anderson's documents over my cardiologist's document. What a blessing! I was so grateful this was no longer an issue.

Now, this book isn't about the healthcare industry or anything, but I am going to say that there is room for improvement for sure.

I'm a huge advocate for listening to our own bodies and speaking up. I wish I would have had the confidence then that I do now when it comes to advocating for myself and trusting my intuition. But that is something I had to learn over time through my experiences.

I think doctors are amazing, and I know they save lives, like mine when I had cancer. But they are also just as human as you and I are, and they make mistakes and misdiagnose people. No one should ever take what they say as fact if they have something inside of them telling them it is not right. Even if you don't know exactly what is going on. In your heart you will know if what a doctor tells you is right or not.

Always listen to that small voice inside you. It's your internal compass guiding you. The white coats don't know everything, sweet sister. Do your research and trust that you know your body better than anyone does.

Tips I've learned over the years:

1. Take someone with you to important doctor appointments. 2 brains are better than 1.

2. Write down your questions and concerns in advance.

3. Have a friend/family member take notes on what the doctor tells you.

4. Seek a second opinion if you are uneasy about a diagnosis.

5. Track your symptoms on your phone. Details. Details. Details.

6. Ask the doctor to repeat herself if you don't understand.

7. Have your pharmacy address and phone number saved in your phone.

8. Always grab your doctors' card. Add all the information to your contacts on your phone.

9. If you have multiple appointments that day, take some snacks, a drink, a book, and something to work on.

10. If you don't vibe with the doctor, get a new one.

Struggles make you stronger and strength fuels confidence.

#upstruggle

Chapter 12
Let them do hard things

"Don't handicap your children by making their lives easy."

-Robert A. Heinlein

I once heard someone at church say this quote, and it has stayed with me over the years. I often think of this with my children when I see them struggling and want to jump in and make everything better. But then I remind myself that I'm not here to make life easy for them. What would that teach them? Not a whole lot. I mean, I'm not trying to make their lives hard, but I'm not rescuing them and trying to save the day either. I want them to learn how to do that for themselves.

If someone always jumped in and "saved the day" when I was struggling, how would I learn and grow? I'm not saying we shouldn't help our children, but I do believe they should try and figure things out, and if they can't, then come to us for help.

I always think back to my struggles and how much they have taught me, and that if I jump in and save the day when my children are struggling, I would be stealing from them the same opportunity my struggles have given me.

I'm here to help them grow up to be well-rounded adults, and they need to experience hard things in their lives for that. Those are gifts, not punishments.

Bubba, my first born son, (no that's not his legal name, but it's the name I gave him when he was a baby, and it's the name I will always call him by) and Ryan went out with some scouts to do a 54-mile hike in New Mexico that lasted for 2 weeks.

I knew this would be tough for them, but I knew it wouldn't kill them. I knew it will build their bond and hopefully teach Bubba some things along the way. But I think it also taught Ryan something too.

When Ryan got home from their trip, he told me about an experience he had with Bubba. On one of the hardest days of their trek, when they had to summit the highest peak, Bubba told him he was struggling to continue due to a blister on his foot. Instead of allowing him to give up, Ryan encouraged him to push past the pain.

Despite the pain Bubba felt with each step he took, he decided to keep going. After another hour of hiking, they could see the summit in the distance. The climb looked scary and difficult to accomplish, not just for Bubba but for Ryan too.

The two made eye contact and together decided to tackle the final ascent. Halfway up the climb, Ryan noticed that Bubba had stopped. It was clear to him just how difficult this was for his son. Bubba was emotional and told Ryan he didn't know if he could make it all the way.

Although very difficult for Ryan too, he pointed to the summit and told Bubba, "You are so close to the finish, it will be hard, but we can do it together." He then placed his hand on Bubba's back and proceeded to push him up the mountain. Now making it twice as hard for Ryan. With renewed strength, Bubba took off and reached the summit on his own. When Ryan reached the summit, Bubba was waiting to embrace him. Ryan let Bubba know how proud he was of him and asked him if it was worth it. He said yes. Together they enjoyed the view.

Ryan told me he noticed a bit of confidence in Bubba the next day as he was talking to the other scouts about summiting.

Mama, I get it! Trust me. We feel like we need to prevent any and all discomfort for our kids. But how will they ever learn and grow if we do that?

Let them do the hard things. Because on the other side of hard, confidence awaits! When faced with another challenge, they will have something difficult to look back on as proof that they can make it through the tough times. And even if they fail at the hard thing, they can learn from it and apply that knowledge to the future. Sounds like a win to me.

I've also learned to give my kids room to make some mistakes while they are young, and the consequences are small.

Yes, we should guide them and teach them and help them make good choices, but, in the end, they always get to choose. This is something I didn't learn till later as a mother. I realized if I was always making their choices for them or making their life easy, when it came time for them to be on their own, would they know how to make good choices? Would they have confidence to do hard things?

Well, probably not! So now is the time to let them start building the choice-making confidence muscle they need. I say the younger you let them learn these things, the better off they will be as adults.

Cheers to letting our kids do hard things!

struggles are
growth opportunities
in disguise.

#upstruggle

Chapter 13
North Star

"All we need is love" is more than a Pinterest worthy quote to hang on our bedroom wall.

Love is more than a feeling; it is an action word.

Last year, for a week, I studied about love from the Bible. Did you know there are over 100 scriptures that talk about love? Crazy, right?!

I don't think I will adequately be able to put into words how powerful love actually is, but I'm going to try.

And of course, it's going to be from my own understanding and what stood out to me in the scriptures.

I want to share with you the number 1 commandment about love (a commandment is a rule/law from God for our own good, even if we think it is limiting, uncool, unfair, silly, old school, etc.) repeated in the Bible.

But first, ask yourself this, why are things repeated? My answer, because they are important, and we need to be reminded of them.

The number one repeat......LOVE ONE ANOTHER......in one way or another, this was said over and over again. The scriptures teach us that we are commanded to first love God and the second is like the first, to love each other as thyself.

Why do you think that is? Why does the Lord command us to love him and each other? I personally believe it is the recipe for keeping us on the straight and narrow path, which leads us back to him.

Loving God will purify our thoughts and actions. When we let love guide us, we produce more love in the world we live in. And yes, the world we live in is hurting. It's hurting bad. I'm not saying we should live in fear. Because that is not love. I'm also not saying that good isn't in the world, because that would be a lie. There is tons of good going on in the world. But there's tons of heartache as well.

And a lot of the time, this heartache, we bring on ourselves. We are really good at doing that. From sulking in thoughts that are not uplifting to behaving in a way that causes heartache because of our poor choices.

So, what about those times when we are truly affected negatively because of someone else's actions? Well, the scriptures say that all things work together for good to those who love God.

For me, that means that regardless, the struggle is for my own good. I can choose to view struggles as "good" when I understand why I have them and have faith in the teachings from the scriptures.

Regardless if these struggles are self-induced, caused by others, or part of life, we can choose to learn and grow from them. Then help others who are walking the path we once did.

The scriptures also say that love rejects and covers all sin! Wait, what?! This one was really big for me. If love rejects/covers all sin, no wonder Satan is everything love is not. And no wonder love is what combats Satan. He uses us against each other. Which is why God says over and over and over again, we are commanded (he does not suggest we love each other or him, he commands it) to love him and each other.

He knew it would be the exact prescription we needed to heal our souls. Love is the key to keeping all of God's commandments! The Bible says so.

Ok, so what is love? We need to understand it so we can apply it. It is patience, kindness, selflessness, clean thoughts, dependable, truth teller and seeker, well behaved, it casts out fear, meekness, slow to anger, does not boast, is not proud, faith, hope, sincere, unity, compassion, tender hearted, respect, so really all the good stuff! More than just feelings, right? I mean, this stuff takes action on our part.

The scriptures also say that we should have faith, hope, and love, but that love is the greatest of all 3. Wow! Faith and hope are a pretty big deal, and if love is greater than those two, then holy moly, that's gold all the way. Maybe there is something behind this whole love thing, huh?

We cannot love God and hate each other. Hating each other means we do not know what love truly is and it means we certainly don't love God. I personally don't believe in the mindset of hating or not liking people. I believe we can dislike people's actions. But disliking them as a person feels wrong to me. Not wrong because that's what's taught in my church but wrong because it doesn't feel right in my heart. I believe a person is far more than their choices. I believe hate is a dangerous emotion. I believe if something feels wrong in your heart, you should listen to it.

I also believe we all make poor choices from time to time. Those poor choices look different person to person. Your worth and my worth will never change because of those choices. Your worth and my worth is not something that comes with accolades but simply being a child of God.

This isn't to say we won't find ourselves frustrated with each other. I mean, we are flawed human beings...and news flash, we will be for the rest of our lives, but we can't use that as an excuse to sit in our sins and not even try. I do believe we should strive to do and be better.

Let's not forget that it's a commandment to love others as THY-SELF. That part of the commandment never stood out to me until a few years ago.

I believe if we truly love God, we can learn to love ourselves, and if we learn to love ourselves, we can learn to truly love others.

We cannot love others the way God intended before learning to love him first. In my life, I have found the more I love God and myself, the better I am able to love other people.

If you are ever feeling overwhelmed with all the commandments, may I suggest that you start with learning about love so you can understand what it means and apply it to your life.

And I know this is a lot, so let's talk action steps, shall we?!

1. Learn about love. Study it from the purest source on the earth, the scriptures.

2. Find 1 (start small and add onto it) area of your life where you can apply it. Maybe in your marriage. Maybe in your relationships with your child, mother, sibling, mother in law, etc.

3. Take action now. It might be messy or feel weird at first but keep doing it. With time, it will become second nature, and you won't have to try as hard. Messy action will always beat inaction.

4. Understand that you are not ever going to be perfect in this life. You are a flawed human being just like the rest of us....... but rest assured, my sweet sister friend, you are ENOUGH. Give yourself some grace.

So, I guess it's really true then, all we need is love.

Let love be your North Star, and it will always guide you in the right direction.

Struggles are meant to change you, but how will always be up to you.

#upstruggle

Chapter 14
Till we meet again...

April 8th started off like any other ordinary Monday; the kids went to school, Ryan went off to work, and I went to the gym to teach two fitness classes.

After the gym, I went home to get ready and run some errands, when, to my surprise, my husband is walking into our bedroom. Before I could greet him with my typical hug and kiss or tell him how excited I was he was home early, I knew. I knew something was wrong. You see, in our entire marriage, I've only seen this expression on his face one other time. My heart sank.

Immediately, I asked him what was wrong. No answer. Again, I said, "Honey, what's wrong?!"

He started crying as he told me his dad let him know his brother Nick had passed away.

I quickly wrapped my arms around him as tightly as I possibly could without suffocating him and just held him. He cried. He cried some more, and all I could think to tell him was how sorry I was.

I could see his pain. I could feel his pain. I so badly wanted to take it all away, but I knew I couldn't. I knew this was just the start of his grieving process, and I knew I needed to let him go through it.

As he shifted to the bed and I kneeled at his feet, I asked him what he wanted to do. He said his parents were headed over to his brother's house right now. I asked him if he wanted to go as well.

Off we went on one of the quietest car rides we have ever had together. I drove and held his hand. I prayed that he would feel his savior's loving arms around him. No, I begged that he would. "Please let him feel your love! Please wrap your arms around him like a warm blanket. Please help me stay strong for him."

We arrived at Nick's home; we were greeted by his roommate and the police officer. Ryan was composed enough to ask some questions.

We weren't allowed into his home just yet. But we had already decided we would wait for his parents Ed and Sharlene, his other brother Will and his wife Crystal to arrive so we could enter as a family.

Finally, everyone arrived. We all embraced each other with hugs and tears. I've never seen my mother-in-law or father-in-law cry the way they did. All I could think to do was keep it together for them. Let them cry, let them feel, support them.

As a family, we all walked into his home. Will, Ryan, and Sharlene went into Nick's room where he laid. Sharlene cried. She was sandwiched between her two boys. Not by accident though, they knew they needed to hold her. I stood back witnessing this and let them have their moment. I didn't want to interrupt. As sad as it was, there was also a sweet tenderness I felt watching them hold their mother like that.

You see, it wasn't all tears. We all laughed as well. It went kind of like this, cry, cry, laugh, cry, cry, laugh, cry, cry, smile. Feel bad for laughing but also understand that even in the saddest moments, there was still reason to smile and laugh.

Nick's kitchen was pretty dirty. The guy could cook, but boy, did he also make a massive mess while doing it. Like hello volcano eruption!

While we waited on the funeral home to come pick Nick up, the brothers did Nick's dishes, and we watched. I mean, two men doing dishes together deserves an audience!

Ed and Sharlene's Bishop (also personal friends) and his wife showed up. The funeral home showed up. And a set of missionaries from our church showed up.

It was time. Time for Nick's body to be taken way. Ryan assisted the guys from the funeral home in getting Nick's body prepared to leave. Sharlene wanted to tell Nick goodbye, and Ryan held her once more.

On the car ride home, he told me he wanted to help move his brother's body. He didn't know why, but he just wanted to. I think, in his own way, that was him showing respect and love to his brother, one final time. I believe he needed to do that. As his wife, standing there watching him do it, my heart broke.

Ryan and I hadn't yet told the kids. We didn't want to tell them before we left only to leave them alone for hours. So, we decided we would tell them once we got home. It was late. But we rounded them up. I could tell Fayth knew something was off. She is really good at reading people, and she was reading her father and I.

In a choked-up voice and with some tears, Ryan let them know. They were all sad and cried. I held Fayth and Noah. Ryan held Elly, and Bubba being Bubba, he sat there and cried in silence as his dad put his hand on his shoulder, as if to say, "I'm here, bud."

As a family, we pulled together to lift and support one another. Each dealing with it in our own little way and in the best way we knew how.

One day, shortly after my brother-in-law passed, Noah, my 11-year-old, came home from school all upset. I asked him how school was, and as he threw himself on my bed, he said, "Terrible, mom, just terrible."

I asked him why. He said, "Uncle Nick is dead, and I'm never going to see him again. I went to school all day and have soccer practice tonight. I'm stressed out. It's too much."

As I hugged him, I told him I was sorry he was stressed out and let him know that going to soccer practice would make him feel better. He asked me how it would do that.

I told him he would see his friends and that moving his body will help him mentally feel better.

He didn't buy it! But Ryan and I convinced him to go to practice anyway. It did make him feel better. And a little ice cream never hurts. No, I'm not above bribing.

The following morning, it was my turn to sleep in and it was Ryan's day to get Noah off to school. By the time I woke up, everyone was gone. My plan? My plan was to stay in bed till I had to get up.

My body was sore and my heart heavy.

Being a fitness instructor, I knew the only way to relieve the soreness was to move my body. So, I did just that. I did some cleaning, got the laundry going, went grocery shopping, made my bed, showered, and dropped of lunch to Bubba.

As I got stuck in my thoughts of deep thinking, as I do when I'm alone, I realized being sore was a lot like grief. It hurts, but not moving only makes it worse. The only way to push past the pain was to move my body.

At first, it's really going to suck. There's just no way around that. At first, the desire to move won't be there. That's ok. The point is to keep moving.

This was what I was trying to convey to Noah that day.

Sweet sister, one day, if not already, you will experience losing someone you love, and it's going to hurt. Remember, the pain is part of the process; the key is to keep moving. The pain is a reflection of the love you have for that person. It's a reflection of all the memories made and the longing to make more. It's a reflection of how much you miss them.

One day, that constant ache will start to subside. It will come back from time to time, and some days it will linger longer than you want. When it does, keep moving.

I would like to leave you with some of my brother-in-law's words. He posted these on November 4th of 2018. These words were shared along with a video of our nephews Rylan and Braylin.

He said, "My nephews playing a gripping game of checkers using Halloween candy! It got intense! I've realized there are a lot of life lessons in the game of checkers alone... here are some of them that I picked up on:

1. You always play to the end regardless of outcome.

2. Sometimes you must lose something in order to gain something more valuable.

3. Always be looking at least 3 steps ahead, otherwise your next move may create a disadvantage.

4. Be willing to sacrifice.

5. Even if you lose, you can learn from your mistakes and play better next time."

-Nick Ferrin

You never truly know
the struggle someone is
going through, give
them the benefit of
the doubt, they are do
ing the best they can.

#upstruggle

Chapter 15
This-N-That Part 3

It's not about you

"Tracey, it's not about you," were some of the most powerful words I was ever told.

Yup, those are the words that my friend Ambryn told me when I was complaining about being offended by someone at church. A true friend is willing to say things that may not always feel good to hear, but because they care, they are willing to say them.

I've learned a lot about being offended. Want to know why? Because I was a pro at it! Yup, like expert style. I was the person who could be offended by the simplest of things. She didn't say hi to me. She didn't look at me. She was rude. She ignored me on purpose. Blah blah blah!

The thing is, it was so dang exhausting!! I decided I wanted to be someone who was no longer easily offended. So, I started to learn about it and changed my perspective.

Here's what I've learned:

1. Most people don't try to offend others. Most people have good hearts.

2. Being offended is one's own insecurities surfacing. It's pain that has never fully healed.

3. Fear can also trigger being offended. "She didn't say hi to me." Well, she isn't the issue; you needing to be liked and worried she may not like you because she didn't say hi, is the issue.

4. It is so much easier to blame someone else for being offended instead of taking responsibility for our own feelings. Being offended

means layers need to be peeled back to the underlying cause of those hurt feelings.

5. Being offended is always a choice. This one was huge for me. I'm all about choices! And once I found out I had a choice, I started to let things go.

Now, this isn't to say, I would continue to surround myself with people who are rude or plain out mean and just take it. That's not me. I just simply let it go with the understanding that one's own actions are not a reflection of me but of them. One's own actions are a reflection of how much they love and respect themselves. If they aren't kind to themselves, why in the world would they be kind to me?

Then I use common sense and limit my interaction with them. Well, at least that's what my common sense tells me to do. But on a more truthful note, as I started to change from the inside out, I just flat out don't even attract those kinds of people.

And here's a kicker! Most of the time, while we are all upset and feeling offended, the other person has no clue and is moving on with their life. Say what! So, who is the one left suffering? Yup! The one who chooses to take offense.

I also remind myself that people have off days and so do I. I would hope someone would give me some grace. So, I try my best to do the same.

Sure, being offended creeps in from time to time, but now I have the tools to keep it at bay or at least be able to work my way through it. Whereas before, I couldn't. Before, I would hold on to a grudge. And sister, that stuff is exhausting.

It isn't about you, and when you make it about you, it's your own crap getting kind of smelly. Let.It.Go.

Dear mama

To the mama having a hard time letting go, I understand.

The day arrives, we go to the hospital and give birth to our child. All the memories of pregnancy discomfort magically disappear because all we can focus on is that sweet baby in our arms.

That little baby needs you for everything! We get in our minds who and what they will become.

We wonder what kind of personality they will have. Will they be more like their dad or me? We develop hopes and dreams for them.

We want them to grow up to be strong and independent. Someone who has a mind of their own. Who isn't afraid to speak up.

We think we know best the kind of life they need to live in order to be happy.

As they start to grow up a bit, they need and want us less, and for the most part, we are ok with it because let's be real, it's nice to finally have children who are a bit more independent, right?

Who don't need us to wipe their butts, give them baths, or make their meals. They can stay home alone and even babysit their younger siblings. Hello new world of awesomeness!!!

Yeah, life's pretty dang good at this point!

And then it happens......they grow up even more!! Except things are much different now. They are fighting for their independence from us. Insert crying emoji face here.

And we're just not ready to let go. We're just not ready to let them make that transition to adulthood. Because it's hard! I mean, at one point, their very own survival depended all on us.

We wonder if they will make good decisions. Will they be capable of handling "real life"?

But what I'm learning is – it really is *their* life. All we can do as parents is love them for who they choose to be and trust that what we have taught them, is enough.

Who cares if they don't become the person we had envisioned in that hospital bed. It's not up to us to say who and what they should become. It's up to them to decide! Their life is not ours to control.

And just because they don't live the life we do or make the same choices we do doesn't mean they've somehow screwed up. It doesn't mean they are lost. It doesn't mean they have ruined their lives.

It means they are their own person, and it's ok for them to choose what kind of life they want to live, even if it doesn't look the same as ours. And we realize......it's time to let go. Let go of what we want for them and let them be the person they want to be, because it was never our decision to begin with.

Sometimes holding on too tight just makes things worse, let go... trust them...let them feel comfortable being who they want without making them feel like something is wrong with who they want to be. They will figure it out, and the fact that you are this concerned only says you are doing a good job at raising them.

~Sincerely, a mama who is figuring it out as she goes.

"Your children are not your children. They are the sons and daughters of Life's longing for itself. They come through you but not from you. And though they are with you, yet they belong not to you. You may give them your love but not your thoughts. For they have their own thoughts. You may house their bodies but not their souls."

-Kahlil Gibran

Get over yourself

Today, at church, I was able to attend a class called Relief Society; we talked about some changes that have been implemented to a program ran by the women of the church.

We talked about how there is a need and desire for unity and friendship among the sisters (that's what we call each other, yes, we were using the word sister before it was even cool to use) of the church.

Everyone had an opportunity to voice their opinions or experiences with this program and the changes that were made.

When it was my turn, I expressed that in order to create unity and friendship, we need connection. And connection in my opinion is created by learning how to get over ourselves by talking about the things that we try so hard to hide.

You know, those things we feel shame or embarrassment over. Those things that we feel others might judge us for. Those things we try so hard to keep a secret. Yes, those are the exact things that must be talked about to create connection.

You see, sometimes there is this self-imposed pressure in my church to appear to have it all together. I also think this is something a lot of women struggle with as well. Not just church goers.

So many ladies don't talk or openly talk about struggles they are having. And hey, I really do get it. You think it was always easy for me to talk about everything I've shared in this book with you? Heck no!

But it's those very things that we have to talk about to build connection with one another.

News Alert, no one has a struggle free life. It just doesn't exist. You have got to be crazy to think anyone does. Look, some just hide theirs well.

I don't care who you are or what status you hold, you are not exempt from downright nasty trials. The ones that will have you question your faith and purpose. The ones that will drag you through the mud.

Everyone experiences them at some point in their lives. So why hide it?! Why think you are alone?! Why turn inward?! Why feel shame or embarrassment?!

That's Satan's way! He wants us to feel that way. Christ doesn't!! We've got to learn to let go of this fake illusion that we are strong ladies and, as such, we don't need to reach out for help. Because a strong woman doesn't talk about her feelings. A strong woman doesn't ask for help, she gives it. A strong woman can do it all by herself, thank you very much.

No, that's called Satan's way! That's called pride. That's called you haven't learned how to get over your damn self.

I'm not saying plaster your dirty laundry all over social media for the world to see!! Because sister, there is a proper way to talk about the hard things you are going through without whining, complaining, and pulling others down with negative vibes.

But my gosh! Everybody goes through struggles. Yes, those struggles are different from person to person. But the feelings are universal, remember? I talked about this in the intro to this book. Feelings are things we can all relate to. Different story, same feelings.

We don't have to be exactly alike to understand each other. We don't have to agree with each other to show empathy. Heck, you don't even have to agree with everything I wrote in this book to be friends with me.

But we do have to get over ourselves and be brave enough to open our hearts and share our feelings. That's what a strong woman does!

Struggles start off
neutral you get to
choose the meaning
you give them.

#upstruggle

Chapter 16
Love What Matters

When my cancer story went live on the Love What Matters Facebook page, I was taken aback with some of the comments that people were leaving. I mean, after all, this page is called, Love. What. Matters. I just poured my heart out through my story, and all some readers could focus on was the one aspect of my ex leaving me when I was sick. An aspect that only got one paragraph. A paragraph that was in no way bashing or opening it up for the comments received.

Comments like:

"How dare he leave you sick and pregnant."

"What ever happened to in sickness and health?"

"She's better off without him."

"What a jerk."

"Think about the message he is sending those girls."

It got to the point that I had to stop reading the comments because I was getting upset.

The message I hope my girls take away is that people make mistakes, all people. Yes, sister, even you and me.

That he loved them so much he was willing to sign over his rights because he knew he couldn't take care of them the way they deserved.

That we all do the best we can with what we have and that when we know better, we do better.

That their mom is no victim to anything or anyone.

That love truly can heal a broken heart.

That no matter what struggles come their way, what they choose to do with them is and will always be their choice.

That their mindset matters. What they believe matters. I want them to know that forgiveness is not for the other person but for themselves, so they can move forward.

I refuse to be on the bashing the ex-bus, that bus is headed the wrong direction and nothing good can come from it. Surely, those who only read my story but didn't live it can see the silver lining too.

I choose to have a perspective that is healing. One that adds value to my life. One that brings peace and love to my soul.

If you ask my girls, they will tell you that I have never bad mouthed their biological father to them, not even once. In my eyes, bashing their biological father would be completely selfish of me. Talk about sending my girls the wrong message. What kind of message would that send them? How do you think that would make them feel? What kind of example would that be setting?

I choose to not have a victim mindset. I choose to not hold onto negative energy. Saying unkind things about my ex just doesn't make me feel good.

What those people who made those unkind comments didn't know, was in 2015 I received a phone call from my ex-husband's father, informing me that my ex had passed away the day before. I shut down and didn't know how to feel or if I had the right to feel anything at all.

I had been at a point in my life for many years where I only wanted him to be happy in his life. When I was able to come to that place, I knew I was in a good spot. I saw him as a son of God and knew his worth was as great as anyone's. Even if he didn't always make the best choices, that never changed his worth. I knew that.

It wasn't till that next morning that his death hit me, and it hit hard.

I worried about showing my true feelings over his death to my husband. Worried somehow Ryan seeing me cry over the loss of the man I was once married to, would hurt him. I didn't want to hurt him, but I should have known better. Ryan held me many times and wiped away the tears of heartache, I cried over the loss of another man.

He gave me blessings of comfort that were beyond tender and sweet. He told me it was ok to be hurt, and that although he didn't share the same feelings, he understood.

He showed me Christ like love beyond what I ever thought possible. Together with our girls, we attended my ex's funeral. I felt like no one could understand how I was feeling. My feelings seemed so complex. Then I remembered there is always one person who knows the pain I felt. The Lord and Savior, Jesus Christ.

Struggles are not an excuse to give up, they are a reason to keep going.

#upstruggle

Chapter 17
Heart work over Hard work

Communication has been vital in my marriage! This was something I didn't always understand early on in our relationship, nor was I good at it.

When I would get frustrated with my husband, I wanted to be left alone, but he wanted to talk. Talk? Are you kidding me? That was the last thing on my mind. Like, just let me sit in silence without you trying to talk things through like a mature human being and let me sulk over why I'm upset. Because that always made me feel better... said no one ever.

I may not have been great at communicating with him when we first got married, but I knew I wasn't going to start a habit of saying things out of frustration or anger, only to regret what I said, later. He knows when I do say something, it's because I mean it. We'll never leave each other guessing where we stand or how we feel. If our facial expressions and actions don't convey it, our words will.

Ryan expressed his frustration with me as we sat in the hot tub tonight; his frustration came from not meeting the frequency of how often he wants to have sex. If I'm being honest, I wasn't caught off guard by this conversation. I knew it was coming. Because it's the conversation we've had multiple times throughout our marriage.

Physical touch is one of my husband's top love languages. And here's the kicker, it's also one of mine. I know this, and he knows this. We both enjoy hugging each other, kissing, snuggling, hand holding, flirting, and SEX, but we both need all those things in different doses. Yes, I'm a Christian girl talking about sex in a book.

I let him know I wasn't trying to frustrate him on purpose, but that I understood his frustration. Because I know how I feel when he's not meeting my needs in the doses I want, and we have to have a conversation about it. I understand where he is coming from, I get it! Who am I to say that what he needs is asking too much of me or not enough? That's not my job. My job as his wife is to know his needs and wants, then try my best to meet them, and when I'm not, be willing to talk it through with him and commit to trying harder. Even if it's a conversation we've had countless times.

As we sat in the hot tub, we talked about the different ways we could meet in the middle. Ways that I could meet his needs but also his willingness to adjust his expectations. We talked about what was realistic in our marriage and that his needs matter, and so do mine. Yes, we even talked about the frequency of how often he wants it versus how often I want it. No, they don't align! For most of our marriage, they haven't.

It's not that I don't love him or desire him. Because I do! I just don't need sex as frequently. We both have had to come to the understanding that it's ok that we are different but that doesn't give either of us the right to not keep trying or expect that it's going to go exactly how the other one wants it to. It's about meeting in the middle. It's about trying harder. It's about showing each other we really do care. It's about being committed and being willing to listen.

We haven't given up on this either. We both know we need to work at it, and because we love each other, we do. Our conversation didn't go perfectly. We have room for improvement when it comes to these kinds of conversations with each other.

But I'm grateful we both feel comfortable with the space we've created between us, to the point we feel we can always talk about things like frustration or not feeling fully connected like we would like to, and how we can get back on track.

We've been married for almost 16 years, and in those years, we've learned a lot about what it takes to make a marriage successful.

And communication, healthy communication is a HUGE part of it. We've learned that attacking each other or pointing the finger doesn't drive change or make an already frustrating situation better. It only creates more tension.

When we have these conversations, we do it in a setting that is calming for both of us, and we talk it out. We don't yell. We don't name call. We don't blame. We simply express our feelings to each other and honor them. And by doing that, we are able to resolve any frustration we may have with one another.

Marriage is one of those relationships that if you want to work and be successful, it needs constant communication and redirecting when it feels off track. Which boils down to consistent work. I believe whole heartedly that marriage isn't meant to feel like hard work, it only feels that way if the wrong work is being done.

The wrong work stems from the head in the form of ego, pride, and selfishness. Whereas the right kind of work will always come from the heart, also known as love.

The right kind of work doesn't mean that there will never be uncomfortable or tough conversations. It means that when both partners do the right kind of work, it will lead to a positive outcome. The wrong kind of work will lead to a negative outcome.

Our conversation of him expressing frustration with me led to us both feeling understood and being affectionate with one another. Our marriage has been successful not because we do things perfectly, but because we respect each other, are willing to talk about things that bother us, and course correct when needed.

A marriage will always feel like an uphill battle when the wrong work is present. The moment the wrong work is cut out, that clears room for heart work. And when heart work is in a marriage, it will be successful.

"Marriage is a gift from God to us. The quality of our marriage is a gift from us to Him."

-L. Whitney Clayton

Struggles are a compliment from a loving God who believes so fully in you that he is allowing you to go through this.

#upstruggle

Chapter 18
Not again!

Remember that podcast Empower HER I told you about? Well, I actually met Kacia through a company called Beachbody. We shared the same upline coach. And that retreat I went on, she was on it too. I had that "you're too cool for me and would never want to be my friend" high school moment when I saw her for the first time.

This girl was confident, happy, and outgoing. All the things I admired about other people and was working on being myself.

Anyway, Kacia had a girl on her team named Brittany. Now, I never met Brittany in person. I only found out about her through social media in 2018 when I came across a post Kacia made about her having ovarian cancer. Britany was on the brink of death, and it was her dad who actually mentioned ovarian cancer to her doctor. She was 27 and married when she was diagnosed, and it wasn't till she had gone through 12 doctors that the 13th one found what was wrong with her. Then, she was diagnosed with breast cancer, while fighting ovarian cancer. #nowords

I started following her on Instagram. I was so impressed with how she was facing cancer head on and not letting it steal her joy. Which was the complete opposite of what I did when I was sick all those years ago. Back then I didn't have the tools to deal with it the way she was. This wasn't to say she didn't have bad days, because she totally did. She just chose to stay positive and looking up.

Kacia made a post on her Instagram account back in May of 2019, and said she had a gut feeling that she needed to bring Brittany on her podcast right away because she felt it would save a life. When I read that, for some reason it resonated with me. I felt like it was for me. But then again, I was like, but I don't have ovarian cancer, so how could it be for me?

I hopped on over to her podcast, where episode #48 with Brittany was waiting for me. I listened to it and again had that strange feeling it was for me. But how? I don't get it. This made zero sense. I kept this in the back of my mind and went on with life.

Starting to make sense

"I feel off. I'm not saying anything major is wrong with me, it could be minor. I don't know. I just know something is off."

That's what I had been saying to my friends and husband for several weeks.

Their response?! "Tracey, you're getting older." And I'm like, whatever! I'm not that old. With everything I had already been through and knowing that I am very in tune with my body, I decided to schedule an appointment with my doctor to see if we could figure it out. She quickly diagnosed me with perimenopause.

I mean, did I even spell that right?! That certainly wasn't on my radar or even part of my vocabulary yet! I thought I had another 10 years before I had to worry about anything like that.

Talk about shock. But then again, with everything I had already been through with my health, it just seemed like one more thing. So, was it really that surprising? Not really.

It's frustrating, for as long as I can remember I feel like I've had to fight for my health. Something I hadn't mentioned yet is that I also have stage 3 chronic kidney disease. Just admitting that makes me feel sick to my stomach. We keep an eye on it, and for many years, it's been stable.

I feel like my body, to some degree, isn't mine. My mind says, "Tracey, you are strong and, oh, so healthy." Then sometimes, my body just laughs in my face and tells me I'm not. My health is a sensitive topic for me. Not because I'm embarrassed. I'm an open book and transparent.

But because having to admit that my health isn't 110 percent is HARD. For a girl like me, who likes to take ownership of her life, to admit that she doesn't always have control over her own health, is a struggle.

After sitting on my new diagnosis, I realized the reason I was so quick to accept it wasn't because I agreed with my doctor. It was because I was relieved it wasn't anything she was concerned about or anything that warranted further testing.

She seemed so sure that perimenopause was what I was dealing with, that even when I told her about the constant cramping and back pain, she quickly whipped out a calendar, asked me when my last period was, dragged her finger two weeks out from that date, and said, "You're ovulating and that causes cramping." No duh! But this much? That much cramping was not my normal.

Over the next few days, I had this nagging feeling that she was wrong, and perimenopause wasn't what I was dealing with. I kept thinking about Brittany and her story and how she was misdiagnosed, and no one would listen to her or told her it was all in her head. I also thought back to when I was misdiagnosed with that heart condition, and even though I didn't know it at the time, I had that same nagging feeling that something was "off."

This nagging feeling grew stronger, so strong that I woke up at 2:30 am one morning and hit up the research hard core. I even listened to episode #48 again.

Knowing Brittany's story and how she was misdiagnosed multiple times before getting the correct diagnosis, gave me the boost of confidence I needed to seek a second opinion and not feel that I was overreacting.

That morning, I set up another doctor appointment with a different doctor to get that second opinion. Because if there is one thing this girl has learned over the years, it's to not ignore her own feelings. Especially the ones that won't go away. I'm not perfect at it, but I do try my best to listen to them.

My new doctor agreed; she too didn't think that what I was dealing with was perimenopause. She recommended that I get a pelvic ultrasound done and make an appointment to see a gynecologist to get the results. She said this was outside her scope of practice but definitely doesn't think its perimenopause.

I did my ultrasound Friday after I taught my class. My bladder was full, and I was ready to go. The technician was super kind. I was there for a transvaginal ultrasound, have you done one of those before? She held up this large wand and told me to insert it into my vagina just like I would a tampon. My eyes got really big, and I told her lies all lies and that it's definitely not like inserting a tampon. She laughed and told me she really needed that. We were just like two girlfriends having a conversation talking about things girlfriends do, all while she was probing my vagina taking pictures. I mean, no biggie.

I figured since this wasn't my first rodeo that I would be able to read her. Most technicians can't help themselves. Their heads start to tilt, they squint their eyes, or they focus on one area longer than others. I'm sure they are trained to keep a poker face, but after all, they are human, not robots.

This lady showed zero signs on her face that anything was wrong. Oh, her poker face was good!

That same afternoon, my phone rang, and my doctor was on the other end. So much for making an appointment to get the results! You know it's never good when the doctor calls you and uses words like complex, stat, and concern.

She told me I had some fibroids in my uterus. But that's not what concerned her. She then began to tell me that I had 2 cysts on my ovaries. She called them complex cysts. I asked her what complex meant, and she said a cyst with shadowing. Like I have any idea what that means. But I knew I would hit up the internet as soon as we got off the phone to learn more about it. She then began to tell me that the one on my left ovary was small but the one on the right ovary was large, and that's the one she was concerned about.

She told me she wanted me to see her gynecologist, stat. And that if this was going on with her this is who she would want to see for it.

This was on a Friday. I had to sit on this for an entire weekend. Oh my gosh, are you kidding me? Nope. That weekend felt like an eternity. I thought about Brittany again. I thought maybe this was why I felt that post and episode #48 was for me.

I turned to the internet to learn more about a complex cyst. What I found was not comforting and scared the living daylights out of me. I know, I know, everyone always says not to hit up the internet when something like this is going on, but I find it very helpful and read from reputable medical sites. Doing research was something I needed to do. I didn't want to be caught off guard or not be able to follow along and understand what the doctor was talking about.

Who do I talk to?

I thought I was being brave. I thought I was saving others from getting all worked up. I thought I was being selfless.

I didn't want anyone else to feel the way I was. My emotions were all over the place. From feeling fine to feeling like a huge mess. I kept thinking about my struggle formula and the reminders. Especially the one that says, you are not meant to go through this alone. Who are you leaning on that is helping you get through this? Um, me, myself, and I.

Ryan was out of town on a hunting trip with his dad. He didn't have good reception; I had only received a few texts from him while he was gone. He wouldn't be getting home till Sunday. Calling him wasn't an option. Plus, I didn't want to worry him; he was 14 hours away and that would have made his trip home unpleasant for him because he would have worried. I also knew he would have also cut his trip short and come home early.

If there was something seriously wrong with me, that would probably be his last trip for a while, and I wanted him to enjoy it. Right or wrong, that's just how I felt.

Who else can I lean on that I trust? Who else will make me feel better the way he does? Well, no one will ever be as good as he is, but my mom is the next best person. I sent her a text that said, "What are you doing today and tomorrow?" When what I really wanted to say was, "I need my mom. Can you come stay with me till tomorrow?"

But I didn't want to worry her either. She responded to my text and told me she was working till 5, going home to make dinner for the kids, and then take them to look at Christmas lights. She asked me why I wanted to know and what was going on.

I didn't respond right away. I didn't know what to say. She sounded busy, so maybe I should just let her do her thing. You see, my mom is raising two of her grandchildren and also watches a few more while their mom, my sister, is in school and working.

My mom has a full plate, and I didn't want to make her plate any fuller. I know how stressed out she can get with everything she has going on. And I don't blame her, it is a lot. She also works and is in school too. I can only imagine her load.

When I didn't respond back to her, she called me and left a message. My mom knows me well. She knows that when I need something, I need something. She knows I'm not one to overreact or freak out unless there is cause to.

I finally responded to her text message. I told her I wasn't feeling well and wanted to get Noah out of the house. Not all a lie. I asked her if he could go with them to look at Christmas lights.

I couldn't bring myself to say something to her because she knows first-hand how scary cancer is, and I didn't want to worry her. She has had it, she took care of me when I had it, her brother died from it, and her dad (my Papa) died from it. Cancer everywhere, I tell ya!

Here I am, writing a book about struggles and giving tips that I use when I'm struggling, yet for this one, I just couldn't take my own advice right away. I knew I needed to allow myself to work through my emotions before bringing others into my space. That's ok.

I decided to hop in the shower because I knew it would make me feel better and I would stop feeling sorry for myself. I took my phone into the bathroom and played some Christian music from Pandora. Peace washed over me, and I did start to feel a little better.

Ryan called me Sunday morning to catch up and let me know what time he would be home.

I hadn't spoken to him once while he was on his trip, so it was nice to hear his voice again. He asked me how the doctor appointment went and what they said about the ultrasound. I decided to tell him but didn't want to worry him, so I downplayed the anxiety I had over the whole ordeal and made sure not to use any words that would alarm him in our conversation.

He said, "Well, I guess we can't worry if we don't know anything, right?" Bless his sweet soul.

Can you tell he is a man who has never had any major health issues before? Little did he know the entire weekend his woman was in tears and worried sick. I also know his response was due to my delivery of the whole thing, so I don't blame him for responding that way.

It wasn't till he got home that I let him in on everything the doctor told me and the research I had done.

The C word

When Monday arrived, I called to make an appointment with the gynecologist my doctor recommended. The nurse over the phone tried setting my appointment for January 20th. We were in December, a week before Christmas, so I let her know that wasn't going to work because my doctor told me to see her stat.

She told me she would run this by the doctor and see what she recommends I do. When the nurse called me back, all of a sudden, they were able to fit me in the very next day.

The gynecologist said she too was concerned about the large complex cyst on my right ovary. Well, the exact word she used was "suspicious." But who's getting technical over words? I am, the girl who has had cancer before!

She then started using words like, CA125, surgery, staging, ovarian cancer, rupture, severe pain, ER, ovary torsion. All words I was familiar with due to all the research I had done over the weekend.

She said that regardless, the complex cyst had to be removed and referred me to a gynecologic oncologist nearby. But your girl only trusts one hospital for something like this, yup, MD Anderson Cancer Center. I told her that's where I would be going.

I headed downstairs to do blood work like the CA125 test they run for ovarian cancer.

I could feel the tears coming but didn't want to lose it. Now, I don't mind crying. But I knew if I let those tears out, that was opening the flood gates and there would be no closing them. I didn't want those stares from people I didn't even know. You know, the ones that say, what's wrong with her, is she ok, did she just get bad news, or is she crazy and just having a mental breakdown in public?

As I was waiting to be called back for blood work, I texted my husband and told him that he may want to come home early because we would need to call MDACC to get me in. He asked me if I could talk, and I told him no. I was doing blood work and needed to keep my sh*t together and would call him when I was done.

You want to know what I kept repeating over and over and over in my head? "Tracey keep your sh*t together." Cusser or not, which I'm not a huge one. It helped me!

I was even able to call my studio manager to fill her in and let her know I would not be teaching my class that night.

I was dang proud of myself for being able to keep my wits long enough to do blood work and make those two phone calls. I mean, on the phone I did cry a little but not in a hysterical way or anything.

When I got home, I called my mom. I figured it was time to let her know what was going on. I started the conversation terribly by saying, "Don't freak out or anything, ok?" Promise me you will never start a conversation like this. Of course, she said, "Are you ok?" And the tears started. I recounted everything to her that I had been dealing with. No matter how old you get, a girl always needs her mama.

When Ryan got home, we called MDACC to get the ball rolling.

Angry as hell

Being angry isn't an emotion I have very often. Like hardly at all. Most of the time when I'm feeling sad or frustrated, I'm able to quickly flip it around and put things into perspective.

Christmas Eve morning I was angry. Like all-out physically angry. I'm sure my husband could see the steam coming from my ears and most definitely saw the horns peeking through.

I wanted to yell at the top of my lungs and throw a tantrum like a 2-year-old. But instead, I turned some music on and cleaned my house like a madwoman. Ok, I may or may not had gotten some attitude with my husband and son. Hey, my house was sparkly clean! You could have dropped food on my floor and eaten it with confidence.

I went upstairs to my room and caught a glance of myself as I walked past my mirror. I was so shocked with what I saw that I backed up, did a double take, and moved in closer. The girl I saw staring back at me was a girl I hadn't seen in years. She was angry, exhausted, and her eyes sad.

What happened to the woman who glowed with confidence, was happy, positive, strong, and had the attitude of, "bring it!" It's like overnight she was gone.

Then this sweet face walked into my room, and I couldn't help but smile and get excited. That face was my 2-year-old niece. My heart softened, and my attitude quickly shifted. I was able to laugh and smother her with hugs and kisses.

I needed someone to love on me who didn't look at me with worried eyes. I needed someone who still saw me and not what could be. I needed her and didn't even know it till I saw her. Her pure sweet soul was just the prescription I needed.

Sometimes I think she was meant for me. God just knew my sister needed her more, so he sent her to my sister. She even looks like me! But don't feel bad for my sister, Fayth looked just like her when she was younger.

As the fog started to lift, and I was able to see a bit clearer, I was able to reflect a little. I was able to grasp a better perspective on everything because I was no longer marinating in fear.

I want to share a few thoughts with you that I had through my reflection.

1. Allow yourself to feel the feelings that surface. Work through them. Doing this will allow you to process everything you are feeling.

2. No one gets to tell you how you should feel. Everyone experiences things differently.

3. Let others pray for you. Why wait till things are really hard and you're suffocating to let people know what's going on? They can't pray if they don't know.

4. Hold on knowing that eventually the clouds will start to part, and the sun will shine again.

5. Journal your thoughts and feelings. Get them out. I have done this the whole time during this experience, and I'm so glad I have.

6. When you feel ready, do small acts of service for other people. Don't force it. Wait till your heart is ready and you genuinely want to do something.

7. Talk to someone who knows how to listen. Talk them into a coma.

8. Cry. And cry some more. It's therapeutic. "Better out than in, I always say." -Shrek

9. Don't kid yourself into thinking there is only one way to deal or that there is a right way or a wrong way to handle a tough situation. There are multiple ways, and whatever feels right to you is right for you.

10. Surround yourself with people who love you and support you. Everyone else can suck it. Lol...kidding, but not really!

Sense of humor anyone?

January 2nd rolled around, and Ryan and I headed to see the gynecologic oncologist at MDACC. We had to be there so early that no one else was in the waiting room but us. Heck, it was still dark outside.

I'm all about breaking the seriousness that surrounds places like that. I told my doctor that I would try not to pee (I felt like I needed to pee more frequently) on him while he did the vaginal exam. While he was doing the exam, I told him that if I peed on him. He totally deserved it! He laughed and apologized. I mean, there my husband was sitting off to the side and another man (not much older than us) had his hands in my lady parts. Can we agree that the situation needed some inappropriate jokes?

My doctor ordered some blood work and an MRI. He confirmed what my other doctors had been telling me. The only sure way to know if it's cancer we are dealing with or not is to remove the complex cyst and do a biopsy.

On the way home, I texted my in-laws to let them know what was going on. My mother-in-law asked me if I liked my doctor. My response, "Well, I did before he stuck his finger in my butt hole!" I make her proud.

Again, so inappropriate. But like I said, there is no right way or wrong way to deal with a situation like this. This is how I deal with it. I make jokes. And sometimes, really inappropriate ones.

My gynecologic oncologist called a few days later with the results of the MRI; he said that the cyst did look benign and that he would still do a biopsy to confirm it. I was so relieved! He told me he would attempt to do laparoscopic surgery to remove my right ovary, which would only leave a few scars, and that the recovery would be easier and quicker than cutting me open. Of course, it would all depend on once he was in there and how it all goes, as to what he ended up doing. At this point in my life, I don't care about having scars. I've got so many already, what's a few more.

As I waited for my surgery date to roll around, I got my house in order, so I wouldn't have to worry about it while I was recovering. I even gave one last speech and continued to teach my group fitness classes.

Preop with Tracey

Nurse: You may get constipated after surgery.

Me: Oh, I will, I always do after a surgery.

Nurse: You can take stool softeners, MiraLAX, or if you have to, an enema. Do you know how to do an enema?

Me: My husband does. And if I have to do one of those, he can have fun with that...lol.

Nurse: They will remove the ovary through your vagina.

Me (my heart skipped a beat): What!? I thought he was going to remove it from my stomach?! How would he remove it from my vagina? Does he pull it through the cervix? Wouldn't he need to dilate my cervix to do that?

Nurse: No. He would make an incision on the inside of your vagina and pull it out.

Me: No freaking way! Are you kidding me?

Then the fellow who will be assisting my doctor enters the room.

Fellow: Your cyst is the size of a grapefruit.

Me: What?! I thought it was the size of a lemon.

Fellow: Now we're talking about fruit.

Me: Well, a lemon and a grapefruit are two different sizes, so yeah!

Me: Why do you need to take my whole ovary? Why can't you just remove the cyst?

Fellow: Well, the cyst is so big that it's taken over your entire ovary. It's going to be hard to tell the difference between your ovary and the cyst. It distorted your ovary.

Me: So, kind of like having a baby! They grow so big they distort your tummy.

Fellow (perplexed look): Yes, kind of like that.

Fellow: For about 30 mins, while your sample is sent to pathology, we will just hang out in the OR and wait for the results.

Me: So, what? You going to take some selfies with me while I'm passed out on the table?

Fellow (as serious as all get out): Oh, no. Here at this hospital, we don't do things like that.

Me: It was a joke...just a joke.

Me: The nurse said you would have to access my vagina to remove the ovary. Is this true?

Fellow: No. Not for this surgery.

Me: Oh, good! Because I'm on my period...lol... and I was going to say, have fun with that.

The color never returned to his face.

My doctor enters the room.

Me: I told my friends at the gym that you refuse to give me a tummy tuck.

Doctor: Laughs.

Doctor: We are going to try laparoscopic surgery, but if I can't remove the cyst safely or it is cancer, I will need to cut you open.

Me: So, I'm pretty much going to wake up to either a few small incisions or a large cut down my tummy?

Doctor: Yes.

Me: Ok, but when I look down, I better still have two boobs. You can't take those too.

Doctor: Laughs. Yes, those will still be there.

I think my doctor laughed because he has already met me and knows I like to tease, joke, and say inappropriate things. The fellow, poor guy. He seemed so uncomfortable...

Surgery Day

4 am, and the alarm sounded so we could be to MD Anderson by 5:30 am. As Ryan and I were walking the halls of MDACC, I felt peace. I had a man by my side who loved me dearly and whose presence alone gave me the comfort I needed. I was at a hospital that had already saved my life once and that I had full trust and confidence in. IV in, drugs to relax me running through my veins, a few more jokes,

hospital Chaplain preached a prayer, and one last kiss with Ryan before they wheeled me back to the OR. Off to sleep I went.

When I came to, I asked to see my doctor and husband. My doctor couldn't come in right away, but they let Ryan come see me. Because I was so out of it and couldn't lift the blanket to see what he had done to my stomach, I asked Ryan what the doctor told him. He told me his understanding of what the doctor said to him, but my ears needed to hear it from my doctor's mouth.

When Dr. Shafer walked in, I asked him how it went. He said the cyst turned out to be what's called a borderline ovarian tumor. Which is not what Ryan told me, bless his heart. He tried to relay the information correctly but didn't quite get it right. Dr. Shafer said he wanted to monitor me for 5 years because this tumor can come back to my other ovary, and sometimes it can come back as cancer. He let me know that the final pathology report would be ready in about 7-10 days and that when it was, he would call me.

As he was leaving my room, I asked him if my insides were beautiful, and he said yes. Just making sure! Because we all know what our insides look like is far more important than what our outsides look like. Literally and figuratively.

That afternoon I was released to go home. While waiting on the final pathology report, I focused on finishing this book and giving my body time to heal.

My doctor called me today to let me know what the pathology report said. It confirmed I had a Serous Borderline Tumor, also known as low-malignant potential ovarian tumor. It isn't benign because the cells are abnormal but not considered cancer because the cells are not invasive like ovarian cancer. I'm not going to act like I fully understand it, but it sounds like good news to me. He said chemo and radiation were not needed. Can I get a Hallelujah!

What a ride!

Sadly, Brittany passed away at the end of 2019. I am grateful she was willing to share her story with the world. It helped me navigate my own experience and it gave me the extra strength and confidence I needed to seek that second opinion. For that, I am eternally grateful for her. I do not believe the timing of it all happened by coincidence; I believe God had a hand in it. I believe he used Brittany's story to help me and that he will continue to use her story to help countless others. Her story will forever be a part of mine. I wish she could be here today to see how her story has helped me, but I know above, she is aware.

It's been a roller coaster of emotions. All the way from one side of the spectrum to the other. I had some really dark days too. The last time I cried this much was when my Papa died from cancer back in 2011. What I appreciate about this experience is it gave me a renewed outlook on struggles and it only solidified my beliefs about them. This struggle was the shove I needed to #finishthedamnbook. I kept my head down typing on my hardest days. I fully immersed myself into this book and found a strength beyond my own to complete it.

It was important to me to add this chapter. I mean, sure it's easy to talk about a struggle I had 18 years ago and how I was able to work through it over the years. But having to put my formula to the test with a struggle that tied back to that one 18 years ago, was certainly a different experience and just what I needed for my renewed outlook. This struggle was real time. It was happening as I was writing this book. It had the C word in it. It brought a level of fear and emotions I hadn't felt in years. I was forced to truly test my formula out in one of the hardest struggles I have had in a while.

Like I mentioned in the introduction, just because I'm writing this book doesn't mean it's not hard for me to use my own advice. I get that it's not always going to be easy, but at least now you and I have some tools to work through difficult situations.

Some struggles will be harder than others. Some will last longer than others. Some will teach you more than others. Regardless, you have what it takes within you to overcome them. And each time you do, you add another tool to your toolbox. You get to choose the meaning you give them. You get to choose your beliefs about them. You get to choose what you do with them. I pray this book has made you a believer that struggles are for you not against you, if you choose.

Sweet sister friend, I am rooting for you!!!!!

Acknowledgments

Ironically, as I was putting this book together, I found myself needing my struggle formula and reminders more than ever. It's that struggle that gave me the shove I needed to get this book completed. In the pursuit of figuring out how to get my book published, I met Angel Tuccy. She made what seemed impossible, possible. Thank you for showing me the way and for guiding me in getting my very first book published.

Dr. Kane, thank you for being so kind and taking great care of me the way you did. I would not have been able to get into MDACC as quickly as I did if it weren't for you. You will always have a special place in my heart. No doubt we were meant to cross paths when we did. Thank you for not just helping me but also my father in law. You truly are a Ferrin angel.

To my team of doctors (Dr. Robert Benjamin, Dr. Kristy Weber, Dr. George Chang, Dr. Aaron Shafer) and nurses at MD Anderson Cancer Center, thank you for all you do and have done in not just saving my life but the life of others. Future generations are now possible because of your selfless sacrifice in caring for me and all your patients. This book was possible because of you. You truly are angels walking among us.

Dr. Alexander Reiter, you are such a sweet man. I enjoyed having you as my doctor for not 1 but 2 of my pregnancies. Thank you for taking such good care of me and my unborn child when I was sick. You are truly a gifted doctor.

Dr. Gurjit Kaur, I appreciate you so much for taking my concerns seriously and sending me for further testing. I believe patients must trust their doctors, and you certainly have mine. I look forward to continuing to have you as my PCP.

Miguel Guzman, what an honor it was to meet you and work with you. You have such an easy-going happy energy about yourself.

That energy made taking photos for my book so much more enjoyable. Miguel is an award-winning photographer. For more information on how to book him, go to www.mguzanphotos.com.

Brigitte Lindford, you have no idea how much I appreciate you. I am so grateful to you and all the time you took in helping me grow as a human. Thank you so much for investing your time into me. Thank you for introducing me to personal development and believing in me way before I believed in myself.

Heather Palmer Willeby, there will never be another you. Our bond is unbreakable, no matter how many years go by. I love you like a sister and will never forget your loyalty. No one will ever be able to take your place. Thank you for being a true friend to me, especially when I needed one the most.

Ashlie Sustatia, you are so dear to me. It has been a true pleasure to have a front row seat to all your success within the fitness industry. I've enjoyed all our chats before and after class. It's because of you that I'm the instructor I am today. Thank you so much for believing and seeing so much potential in me. I truly adore you!

To my family: my mother, Tracey (Yes, I was named after my mother. She is known as Big Tracey and I'm know as Little Tracey.), my father, Robert, my sisters, Sasha, Kassi, and Porscha. Thank you for all your support during such a difficult time in my life and for loving my girls as your own. Thank you for being such great examples to me on what it means to pull together as a family, what love looks like, the lengths one will go to save a life, and what sacrifice looks like. Special thanks to my sister Porscha, aka Baby, for literally putting her life on hold, moving back home, and being a fulltime aunt to my girls. We couldn't have done it without you.

Ed and Sharlene Ferrin, thank you for raising such a wonderful man. A man that is so perfect for me and who loves me more than I will ever know. Thank you for allowing me to share your last name. A name I am very proud to have.

Nana, I miss you so much. I miss talking on the phone and telling you about everything exciting going on with my family. You loved all of us so well, especially your four babies. If you had a favorite, I never knew because you treated them all like they were your favorite. Thank you for setting such an excellent example to me on how to be a Nana! I miss all your kind and encouraging words. You always saw the glass half full. You always knew exactly what to say to make me feel like a million bucks! I still make your taco salad and goulash for the family. It never tastes as good as yours, but I try. Oh, how I miss your awesome cooking and spending time with you. Till we meet again......

Champions Group Fitness family, what a pleasure it has been to be a part of your lives. Thank you for allowing me to guide you each week in your workouts and for all your support as your instructor. I've enjoyed getting to know each and every one of you. Never forget that you matter and taking care of yourself first makes you a better freaking human being.

To all the Rotary Clubs in the Houston area who have allowed me to come share my story, thank. Keep helping your communities the way you do. No doubt you are changing lives for the better.

LJ Herman with Love What Matters, thank you for pushing me as a writer and for giving me the opportunity to share my story with over 8 million people.

My children, Elly, Fayth, Bubba, and Noah. Thank you for allowing me to be your mother and for making me a better person. Girls, if it weren't for you when I was sick, I wouldn't have felt like I had much to fight for. Elly, thank you for being my caretaker and for loving on me and for pushing my wheelchair. Thank you for kissing my bald head and being such a comfort to me. Fayth, thank you for being a fighter. Thank you for being such a good girl and for always helping out when needed. You are someone your father and I can count on, and we appreciate that about you.

Bubba, you are a strength to our family. You are so much like your father, and I love that about you. Thank you for being all mine for those few short years before you discovered how cool your dad was. Noah, you have been a light to us all. Thank you for loving me so well and for being so kind to me. Never lose your tender soul, it's what makes you so special.

Babe, oh, my sweet babe! Where do I even begin. You have added immeasurable joy and love to my life. Thank you for always believing in me and supporting me. Thank you for loving me so perfectly and putting up with all my crazy. I love that we can be so silly and stupid together. You are so special to me. I appreciate you for being by my side through the tough times. I know I can always count on you. There is no one else I would rather do life with. You are my north star. It's truly an honor to be your wife.

Me, you did it, sister! Never stop listening to your heart; it will always point you in the right direction. Never underestimate your ability to do hard things. Keep being the woman your girls can look up to and the kind of woman you want your boys to marry.

To the reader, thank you for trusting me enough to allow me into your world. I hope you found some really good nuggets in this book that you can apply to your life. I pray you are now a believer that the struggle is for you not against you, if you choose.

About the author

Tracey Ferrin is a motivational speaker, author, and cancer THRIVER. She is also a certified group fitness instructor and enjoys teaching the very classes she took before becoming certified.

Her positive outlook on life is contagious to those who meet her. She is a personal development junkie who loves books, listening to podcasts, attending seminars, or anything that adds value to her life so she can add value to others.

Tracey enjoys connecting with people from all over the world through social media and especially those who are dealing with cancer or living life after it.

She is married to her best friend Ryan, and together they have four children: Elly 19, Fayth 18, Bubba 15, and Noah 11. She lives in Houston, TX with her family. Although not born there, she was raised there and considers herself a Texan.

Before you go

You didn't think this is where we were going to end things, did ya? If we are not connected on social media, let's connect!

Instagram: @TraceyFerrin

Facebook: @TraceyFerrin or @44empowerment

TikTok: @TraceyDFerrin (almost ½ a MILLION followers)

I would love to come speak at your next event! For speaking inquiries, please head to TraceyFerrin.com or shoot me an email: hello@traceyferrin.com

Made in the USA
Middletown, DE
15 January 2021